The Big Book of Stretch Routines

Over 150 different stretching routines, with each routine targeting a specific muscle group or a specific injury.

Walker, Bradley E., 1971
The Big Book of Stretch Routines

ISBN: 978-0-9943733-1-1 (Spiral bound version)
ISBN: 978-0-9943733-2-8 (Electronic book version)

Disclaimers
The exercises presented in this publication are intended as an educational resource and are not intended as a substitute for proper medical advice. Please consult your physician, physical therapist or sports coach before performing any of the exercises described in this publication, particularly if you are pregnant, elderly or have any chronic or recurring muscle or joint pain. Discontinue any exercise that causes you pain or severe discomfort and consult a medical expert.

Cover picture/s supplied by Fotolia and iStockphoto. The Stretching Institute has purchased the non-exclusive, non-transferable, non-sub licensable right to reproduce the cover picture/s an unlimited number of times in online and electronic publications, and web advertisements.

The Stretching Institute™
Website: TheStretchingInstitute.com
Address: 460 Main Ave, Suite 3208
              Wallington, NJ 07057
              UNITED STATES
Telephone: +1 877-580-7771

Contents

Getting Started

I remember the day I saw one of my clients struggling to put together a stretching routine. Sure she had all the stretches right there in front of her, but... Which stretch should she do first? Which one next? How many stretches? It was all too overwhelming!

I realized at that moment I could help her by creating the routines for her. And then all she had to do was pick a routine and follow along.

So here they are: Over 150 different stretching routines that you can choose from. And I've broken them down into routines for major muscle groups and routines for sports injuries. So it's as simple as picking the routine that's right for you and then just following along.

My routines are a little different

One of the first things you'll notice about my routines is that they're a little different from what you're probably expecting: In what way? They only take 10 minutes to complete.

Over the past 25 years I've lost count of how many thousands of routines I've designed for athletes, injury sufferers and health care professionals. And one thing I learnt early on was that including too many stretches in a routine did one of two things.

Either, the client would rush through the routine. Or they wouldn't finish it.

I'm sure you know what I'm talking about: You're looking at a routine that contains 10 or 12 or 15 stretches and you're thinking... *"Even if I just do each stretch twice and spend only 30 seconds doing each one (remember most stretches need to be done on the right side and the left side) it's going to take me forever. I just don't have half an hour to roll around on the floor."*

So that's why I include only 3 stretches in each routine. It gives you a much better opportunity to focus on each stretch; hold each stretch for longer (which is really important); target a specific area instead of trying to cover everything; and be done in about 10 minutes.

How to choose the routines that are right for you

As I mentioned earlier, all the routines have been broken down into routines for major muscle groups and routines for sports injuries. So the hardest job you face is simply choosing the routine that's right for you. How do you do that?

Firstly, ask yourself if you have, or have had an injury that is still causing you problems. If so, start with one of the stretching routines for injuries. You can view the injury list in the contents to find the routines for your specific injury.

A word of caution!
The routines for sports injuries have been designed for injury prevention and/or injury rehabilitation. However, they are not useful (and can even be dangerous) if used during the inflammation phase of an injury, which is typically the first 48 to 72 hours after an injury occurs. This phase can also be identified by increased swelling (or inflammation) around the injury site.

During this phase of the rehabilitation process NO STRETCHING should be used! Stretching during this early stage of the rehabilitation process may cause more damage to the injured tissues.

Avoid stretching during the first 72 hours, or if swelling is still present at the injury site. Use other rehabilitation techniques like rest, ice, compression, heat, massage, ultra-sound, etc. before starting any of the following stretching routines for injuries.

If you don't have an injury, then start with one of the routines for a muscle group. It's not important where you start, but as a general rule; if it's not tight and it's not causing you any problems, you don't need to stretch it. There are a few exceptions to this (such as athletes that require increased flexibility for their chosen sport), but for most people this is a wise rule to follow. So if you perform a stretch and you don't feel any tension in the target muscle group, this would indicate that you're not tight in that area.

As you start to notice which muscle groups are tight and which ones aren't, aim to work on the muscle groups that are most tight.

For example, if you notice that your hamstring muscles are tight compared to your quadriceps, work on your hamstring muscles until you have a good level of flexibility in both.

How to stretch properly

Before starting any of the routines, take a minute to review the picture and read the description of how to perform the stretch.

You'll notice that all the pictures in the routines show the "hold" position of the stretch. So start the routine by slowly moving into the hold position of the first stretch. Once in the hold position it's important to **maintain each stretch for 60 seconds** (each side).

Once the 60 seconds is up, slowly come out of the stretch position and then slowly move into the next stretch (or the same stretch on the other side of your body). Once you've completed all 3 stretches, repeat the routine a second time.

It's important that the intensity of the stretch remains light and relaxed. In other words, don't push the stretch too hard.

To begin with, aim for light tension in the target muscle group. If you feel any pain or severe discomfort, you're pushing the stretch too hard. Back off and reduce the intensity of the stretch until you feel a gentle pull or light tension in the target muscle group.

As your flexibility improves you can gradual increase the intensity of the stretch: But never to the point of pain or severe discomfort.

> *Here's a tip*: Relax and focus on breathing deeply while doing the stretches. Many people unconsciously hold their breath while stretching. This causes tension in the muscles, which in turn makes it difficult to stretch. To avoid this, remember to breathe slowly and deeply during all stretching exercises. This helps to relax the muscles, promotes blood flow and increases the delivery of oxygen and nutrients to the muscles.

For more detailed information on how to stretch properly and how to get the most out of your stretching, grab a copy of the Ultimate Guide to Stretching & Flexibility.

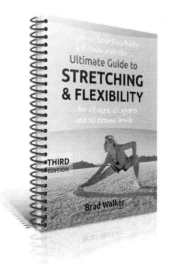

> *Here's another tip*: Cut out all coffee, soda and energy drinks. These drinks are disastrous for your health and especially your flexibility. They affect your nervous system, brain activity and interrupt sleep patterns. They have a dehydrating affect on your body, and not-to-mention, they are highly addictive. If you want to improve your flexibility (and your health), remove them from your diet completely.

My Top 10 All-Time Favorite Stretching Routines

My Top 10 All Time Favorite Stretching Routine #1

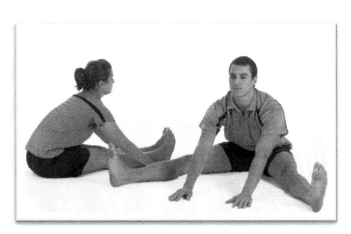

Stretch 1 – Sitting Reach-forward Hamstring Stretch: Sit with both legs straight out in front, or at 45 degrees apart. Keep your toes pointing straight up, make sure your back is straight and then reach forward.

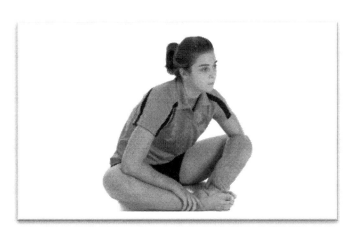

Stretch 2 – Sitting Feet-together Adductor Stretch: Sit with the soles of your feet together and bring your feet towards your groin. Hold onto your ankles and push your knees toward the ground with your elbows. Keep your back straight.

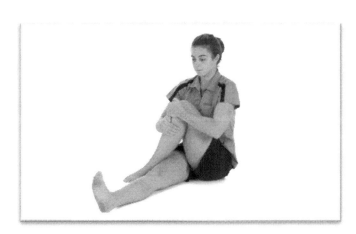

Stretch 3 – Sitting Knee-to-chest Buttocks Stretch: Sit with one leg straight and the other leg crossed over your knee. Pull the raised knee towards your opposite shoulder while keeping your back straight and your shoulders facing forward.

My Top 10 All Time Favorite Stretching Routine #2

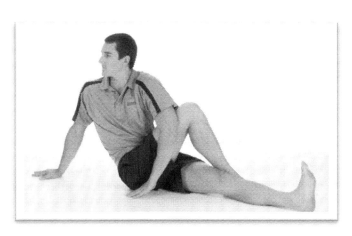

Stretch 1 – Sitting Knee-up Rotation Stretch: Sit with one leg straight and the other leg crossed over your knee. Turn your shoulders and put your arm onto your raised knee to help rotate your shoulders and back.

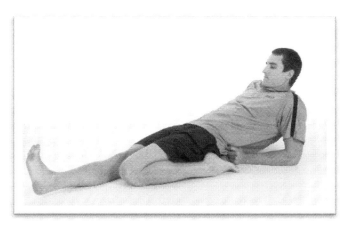

Stretch 2 – Single Lean-back Quad Stretch: Sit on the ground, bend one knee and place that foot next to your buttocks. Then slowly lean backwards.

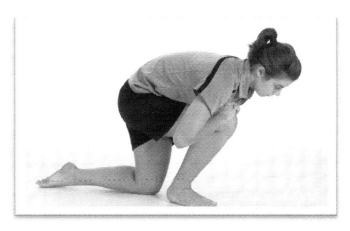

Stretch 3 – Kneeling Heel-down Achilles Stretch: Kneel on one foot and place your body weight over your knee. Keep your heel on the ground and lean forward.

My Top 10 All Time Favorite
Stretching Routine #3

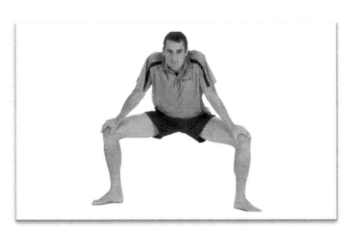

Stretch 1 – Standing Wide Knees Adductor Stretch:
Stand with your feet wide apart and your toes pointing diagonally outwards, then bend your knees, lean forward and use your hands to push your knees outwards.

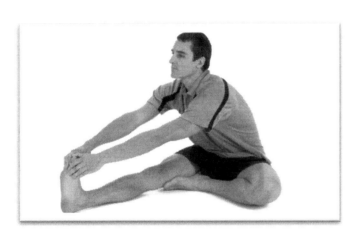

Stretch 2 – Sitting Single Leg Hamstring Stretch:
Sit with one leg straight out in front and point your toes upwards. Bring your other foot towards your knee and reach towards your toes with both hands.

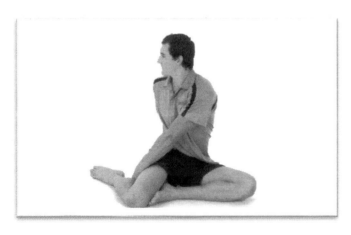

Stretch 3 – Sitting Rotational Hip Stretch:
Sit with one leg crossed and your other leg behind your buttocks then lean your whole body towards the leg that is behind your buttocks.

My Top 10 All Time Favorite Stretching Routine #4

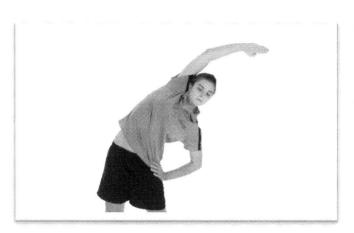

Stretch 1 – Reaching Lateral Side Stretch: Stand with your feet shoulder width apart, then slowly bend to the side and reach over the top of your head with your hand. Do not bend forward.

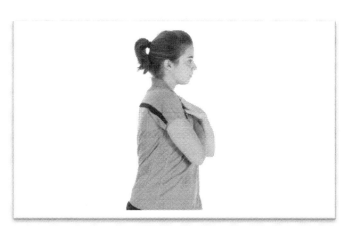

Stretch 2 – Standing Back Rotation Stretch: Stand with your feet shoulder width apart. Place your hands across your chest while keeping your back and shoulders upright. Slowly rotate your shoulders to one side.

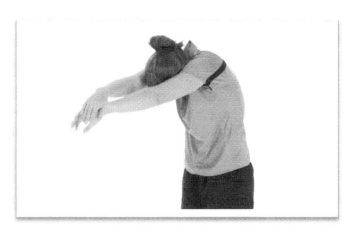

Stretch 3 – Reach Forward Upper Back Stretch: Stand with your arms out in front and your hands crossed over, then push your hands forward as far as possible and let your head fall forward.

My Top 10 All Time Favorite Stretching Routine #5

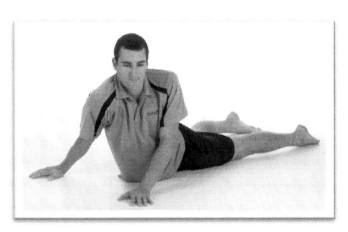

Stretch 1 – Rotating Stomach Stretch:
Lie face down and bring your hands close to your shoulders. Keep your hips on the ground, look forward and rise up by straightening your arms. Then slowly bend one arm and rotate that shoulder towards the ground.

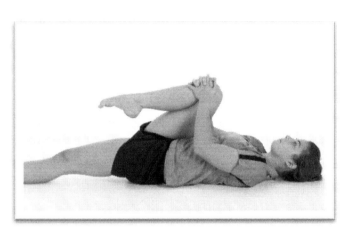

Stretch 2 – Lying Knee-to-chest Stretch:
Lie on your back and keep one leg flat on the ground. Use your hands to bring your other knee into your chest.

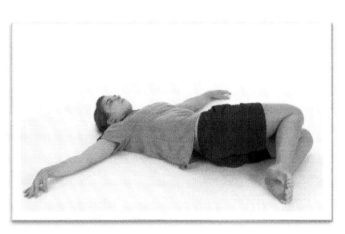

Stretch 3 – Lying Knee Roll-over Stretch:
While lying on your back, bend your knees and let them fall to one side. Keep your arms out to the side and let your back and hips rotate with your knees.

My Top 10 All Time Favorite Stretching Routine #6

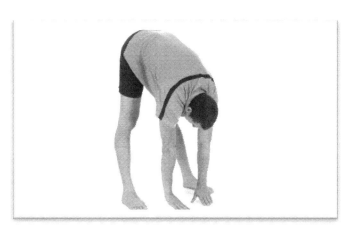

Stretch 1 – Standing Reach-down Hamstring Stretch: Stand with your feet shoulder width apart. Bend forward and reach towards the ground.

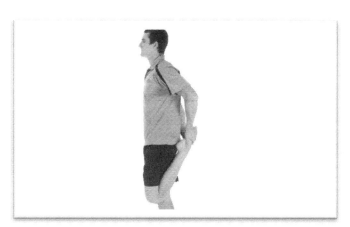

Stretch 2 – Standing Quad Stretch: Stand upright while balancing on one leg. Pull your other foot up behind your buttocks and keep your knees together while pushing your hips forward. Hold on to something for balance if needed.

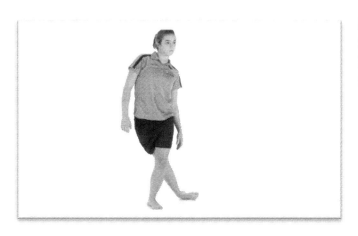

Stretch 3 – Standing Leg-cross Abductor Stretch: Stand upright and cross one foot behind the other. Lean towards the foot that is behind the other.

My Top 10 All Time Favorite
Stretching Routine #7

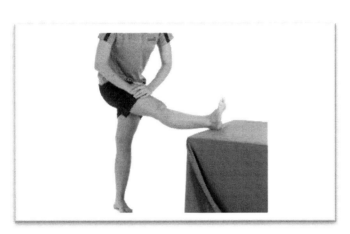

Stretch 1 – Standing Leg-up Toe-in Hamstring Stretch: Stand upright and raise one leg on to an object. Keep that leg straight and point your toes upwards. Then point the toes of your other foot inward and lean forward while keeping your back straight.

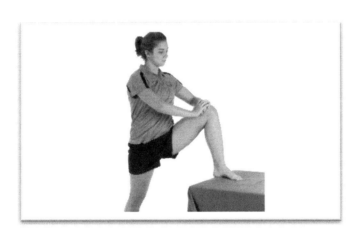

Stretch 2 – Standing High-leg Bent Knee Hamstring Stretch: Stand with one foot raised onto a table. Keep your leg bent and lean your chest into your bent knee.

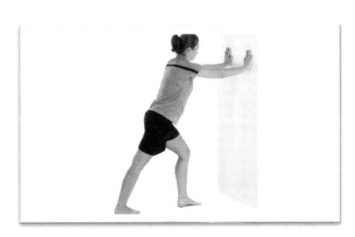

Stretch 3 – Leaning Heel-back Calf Stretch: Reach towards a wall and place one foot as far from the wall as is comfortable. Make sure that both toes are pointing forward and your heel is on the ground. Keep your back leg straight and lean towards the wall.

My Top 10 All Time Favorite
Stretching Routine #8

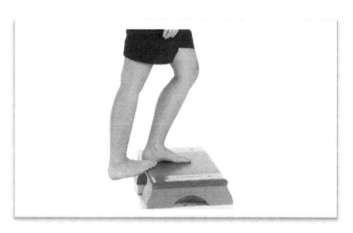

Stretch 1 – Single Heel-drop Calf Stretch: Stand on a raised object or step. Put the ball of one foot on the edge of the step and keep your leg straight. Let your heel drop towards the ground.

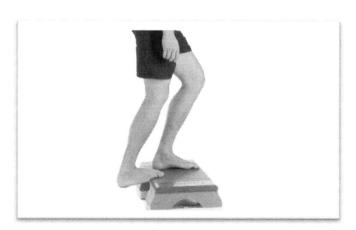

Stretch 2 – Single Heel-drop Achilles Stretch: Stand on a raised object or step and place the ball of one of your feet on the edge of the step. Bend your knee slightly and let your heel drop towards the ground.

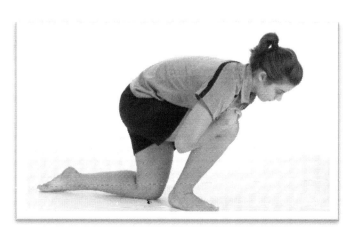

Stretch 3 – Kneeling Heel-down Achilles Stretch: Kneel on one foot and place your body weight over your knee. Keep your heel on the ground and lean forward.

My Top 10 All Time Favorite Stretching Routine #9

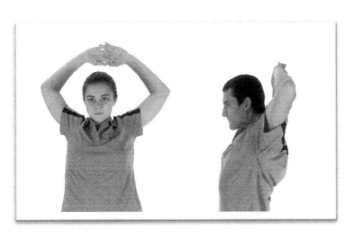

Stretch 1 – Above Head Chest Stretch:
Stand upright and interlock your fingers. Bend your arms and place them above your head while forcing your elbows and hands backwards.

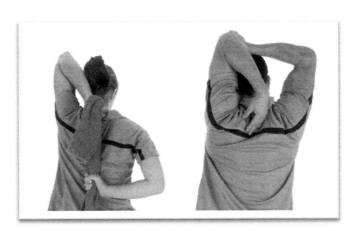

Stretch 2 – Assisted Triceps Stretch:
Stand with one hand behind your neck and your elbow pointing upwards. Then use your other hand (or a rope or towel) to pull your elbow down.

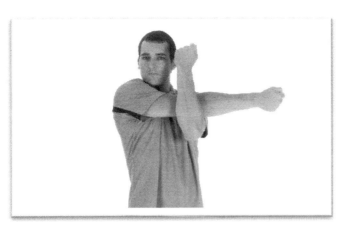

Stretch 3 – Parallel Arm Shoulder Stretch: Stand upright and place one arm across your body. Keep your arm parallel to the ground and pull your elbow towards your body.

My Top 10 All Time Favorite Stretching Routine #10

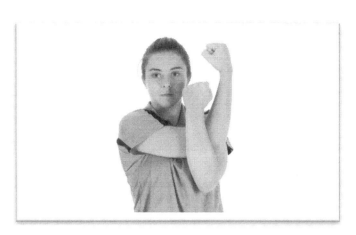

Stretch 1 – Bent Arm Shoulder Stretch:
Stand upright and place one arm across your body. Bend your arm at 90 degrees and pull your elbow towards your body.

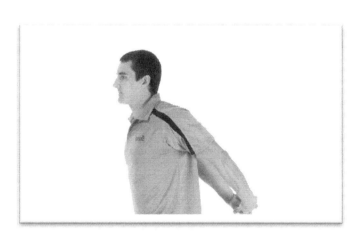

Stretch 2 – Reverse Shoulder Stretch:
Stand upright and clasp your hands together behind your back. Keep your arms straight and slowly lift your hands upward.

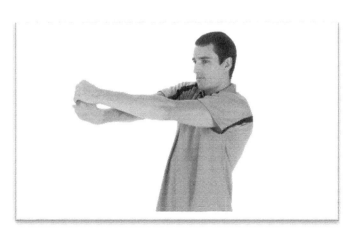

Stretch 3 – Rotating Wrist Stretch: Place one arm straight out in front and parallel to the ground. Rotate your wrist down and outwards and then use your other hand to further rotate your hand upwards.

Stretching Routines for Muscle Groups

Neck Stretching Routine #1

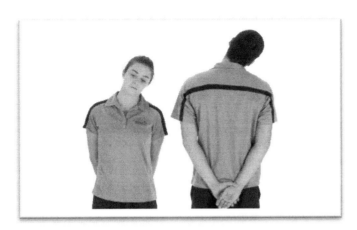

Stretch 1 – Lateral Neck Stretch: Look forward while keeping your head up. Slowly move your ear towards your shoulder while keeping your hands behind your back.

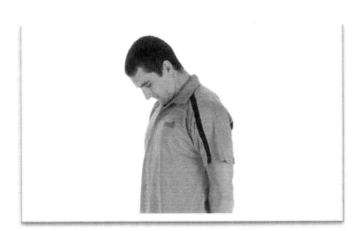

Stretch 2 – Forward Flexion Neck Stretch: Stand upright and let your chin fall forward towards your chest. Relax your shoulders and keep your hands by your side.

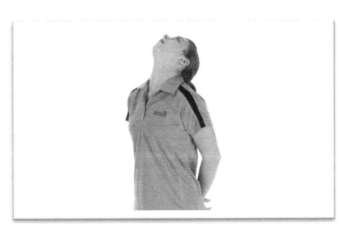

Stretch 3 – Neck Extension Stretch: Stand upright and lift your head, looking upwards as if trying to point up with your chin. Relax your shoulders and keep your hands by your side.

Neck Stretching Routine #2

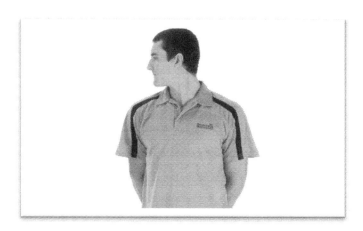

Stretch 1 – Rotating Neck Stretch: Stand upright while keeping your shoulders still and your head up, then slowly rotate your chin towards your shoulder.

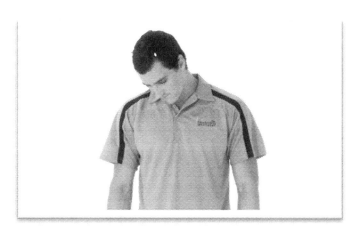

Stretch 2 – Diagonal Flexion Neck Stretch: Stand upright and let your chin fall forward towards your chest. Then gently lean your head to one side.

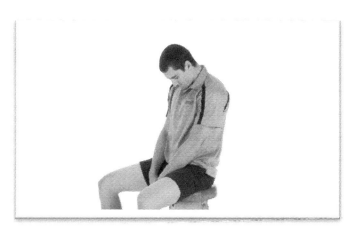

Stretch 3 – Sitting Neck Flexion Stretch: While sitting on a chair, cross your arms and hold onto the chair between your legs. Let your head fall forward and then lean backwards.

Neck Stretching Routine #3

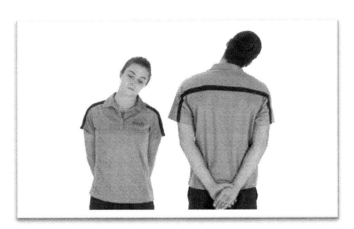

Stretch 1 – Lateral Neck Stretch: Look forward while keeping your head up. Slowly move your ear towards your shoulder while keeping your hands behind your back.

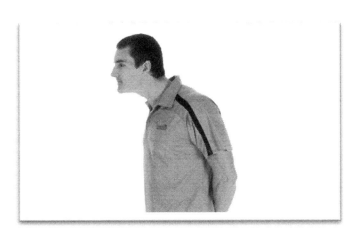

Stretch 2 – Neck Protraction Stretch: While looking straight ahead, push your head forward by sticking your chin out.

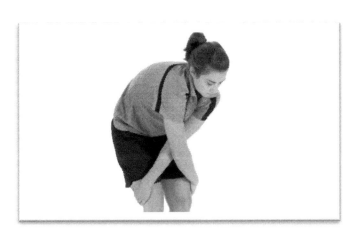

Stretch 3 – Cross-over Shoulder Stretch: Stand with your knees bent. Cross your arms over and grab the back of your knees, then start to rise upwards until you feel tension in your upper back and shoulders.

Shoulders Stretching Routine #1

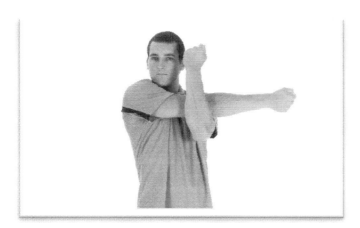

Stretch 1 – Parallel Arm Shoulder Stretch: Stand upright and place one arm across your body. Keep your arm parallel to the ground and pull your elbow towards your body.

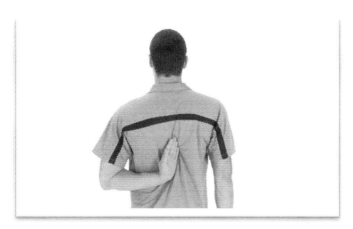

Stretch 2 – Reaching-up Shoulder Stretch: Place one hand behind your back and then reach up between your shoulder blades.

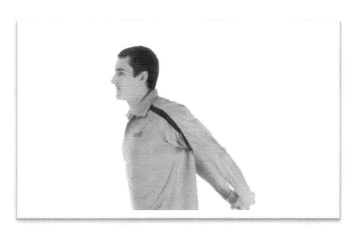

Stretch 3 – Reverse Shoulder Stretch: Stand upright and clasp your hands together behind your back. Keep your arms straight and slowly lift your hands upward.

Shoulders Stretching Routine #2

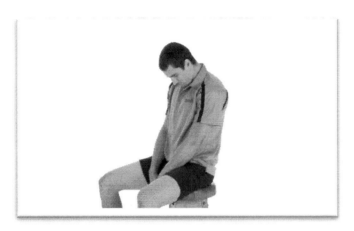

Stretch 1 – Sitting Neck Flexion Stretch: While sitting on a chair, cross your arms and hold onto the chair between your legs. Let your head fall forward and then lean backwards.

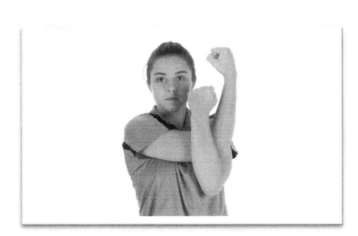

Stretch 2 – Bent Arm Shoulder Stretch: Stand upright and place one arm across your body. Bend your arm at 90 degrees and pull your elbow towards your body.

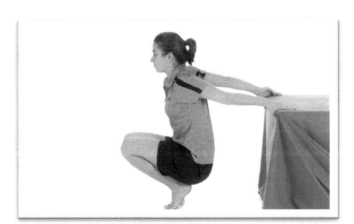

Stretch 3 – Assisted Reverse Shoulder Stretch: Stand upright with your back towards a table or bench and place your hands on the edge of the table or bench. Keep your arms straight and slowly lower your entire body.

Shoulders Stretching Routine #3

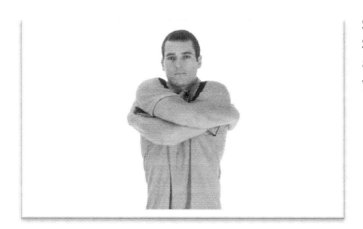

Stretch 1 – Wrap-around Shoulder Stretch: Stand upright and wrap your arms around your shoulders as if hugging yourself. Pull your shoulders back.

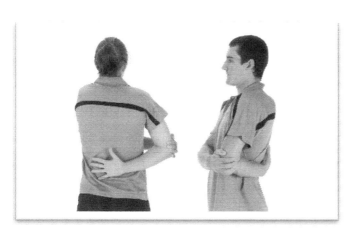

Stretch 2 – Elbow-out Rotator Stretch: Stand with your hand behind the middle of your back and your elbow pointing out. Reach over with your other hand and gently pull your elbow forward.

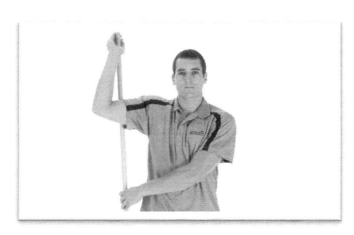

Stretch 3 – Arm-up Rotator Stretch: Stand with your arm out and your forearm pointing upwards at 90 degrees. Place a broom stick in your hand and behind your elbow. With your other hand pull the bottom of the broom stick forward.

Shoulders Stretching Routine #4

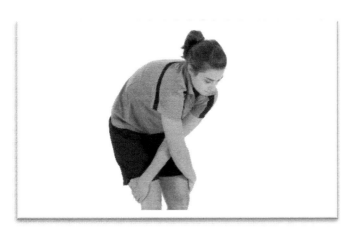

Stretch 1 – Cross-over Shoulder Stretch:
Stand with your knees bent. Cross your arms over and grab the back of your knees, then start to rise upwards until you feel tension in your upper back and shoulders.

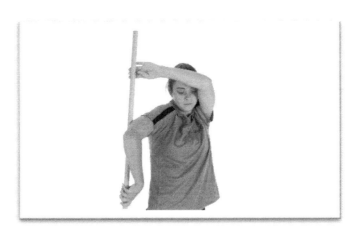

Stretch 2 – Arm-down Rotator Stretch:
Stand with your arm out and your forearm pointing downwards at 90 degrees. Place a broom stick in your hand and behind your elbow. With your other hand pull the top of the broom stick forward.

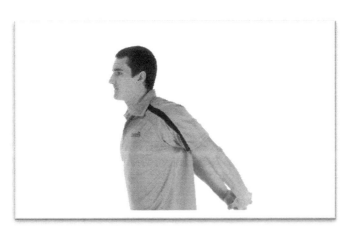

Stretch 3 – Reverse Shoulder Stretch:
Stand upright and clasp your hands together behind your back. Keep your arms straight and slowly lift your hands upward.

Shoulders Stretching Routine #5

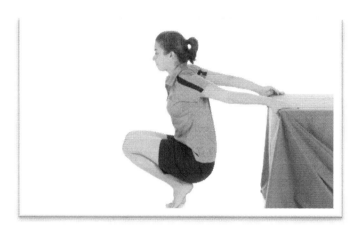

Stretch 1 – Assisted Reverse Shoulder Stretch:
Stand upright with your back towards a table or bench and place your hands on the edge of the table or bench. Keep your arms straight and slowly lower your entire body.

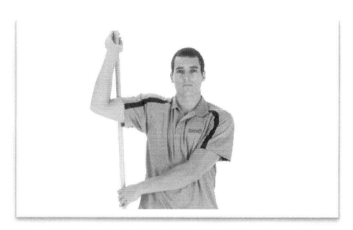

Stretch 2 – Arm-up Rotator Stretch:
Stand with your arm out and your forearm pointing upwards at 90 degrees. Place a broom stick in your hand and behind your elbow. With your other hand pull the bottom of the broom stick forward.

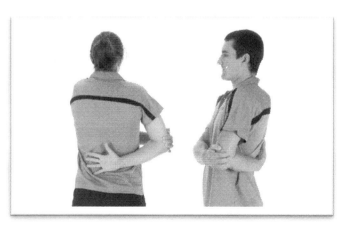

Stretch 3 – Elbow-out Rotator Stretch:
Stand with your hand behind the middle of your back and your elbow pointing out. Reach over with your other hand and gently pull your elbow forward.

Chest Stretching Routine #1

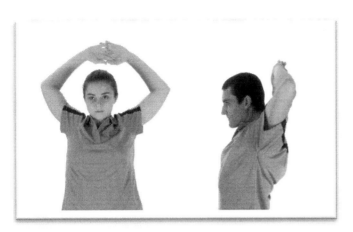

Stretch 1 – Above Head Chest Stretch:
Stand upright and interlock your fingers. Bend your arms and place them above your head while forcing your elbows and hands backwards.

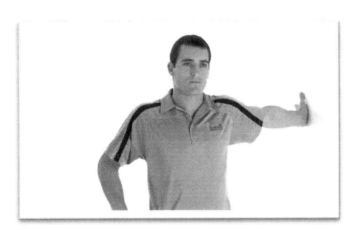

Stretch 2 – Parallel Arm Chest Stretch:
Stand with your arm extended to the rear and parallel to the ground. Hold on to an immovable object and then turn your shoulders and body away from your outstretched arm.

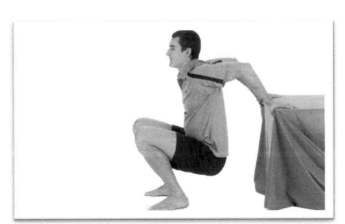

Stretch 3 – Assisted Reverse Chest Stretch:
Stand upright with your back towards a table or bench and place your hands on the edge of the table or bench. Bend your arms and slowly lower your entire body.

Chest Stretching Routine #2

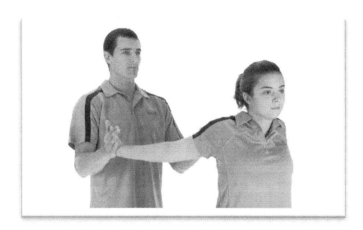

Stretch 1 – Partner Assisted Chest Stretch: Extend both arms parallel to the ground and have a partner hold on to your hands, then slowly pull your arms backwards.

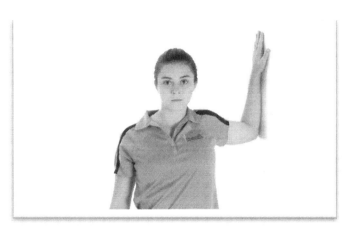

Stretch 2 – Bent Arm Chest Stretch: Stand with your arm extended and your forearm pointing up at 90 degrees. Rest your forearm against an immovable object and then turn your shoulders and body away from your extended arm.

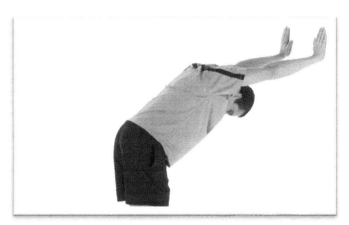

Stretch 3 – Bent-over Chest Stretch: Face a wall and place both hands on the wall just above your head. Slowly lower your shoulders as if moving your chin towards the ground.

Chest Stretching Routine #3

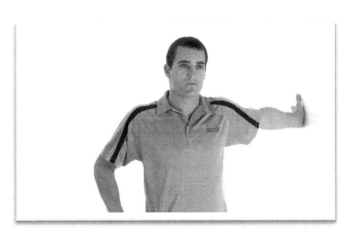

Stretch 1 – Parallel Arm Chest Stretch: Stand with your arm extended to the rear and parallel to the ground. Hold on to an immovable object and then turn your shoulders and body away from your outstretched arm.

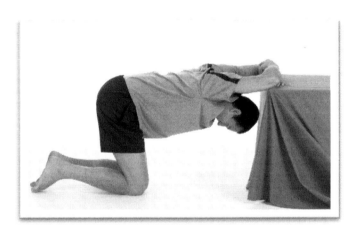

Stretch 2 – Kneeling Chest Stretch: Kneel on the floor in front of a chair or table and interlock your forearms above your head. Place your arms on the object and lower your upper body toward the ground.

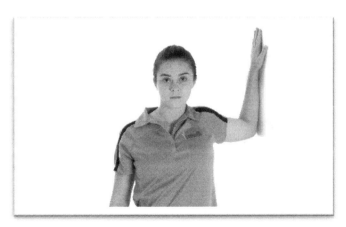

Stretch 3 – Bent Arm Chest Stretch: Stand with your arm extended and your forearm pointing up at 90 degrees. Rest your forearm against an immovable object and then turn your shoulders and body away from your extended arm.

Chest Stretching Routine #4

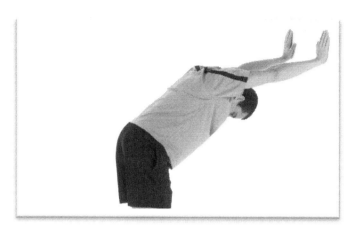

Stretch 1 – Bent-over Chest Stretch: Face a wall and place both hands on the wall just above your head. Slowly lower your shoulders as if moving your chin towards the ground.

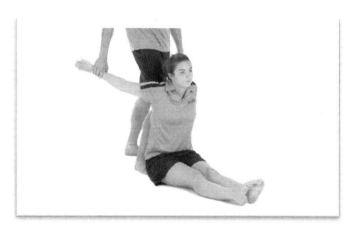

Stretch 2 – Seated Partner Assisted Chest Stretch: Sit on the ground and have a partner stand behind you. Reach behind with both arms and have the partner further extend your arms.

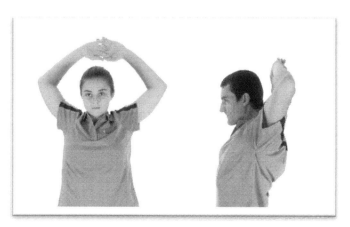

Stretch 3 – Above Head Chest Stretch: Stand upright and interlock your fingers. Bend your arms and place them above your head while forcing your elbows and hands backwards.

Arms & Hands Stretching Routine #1

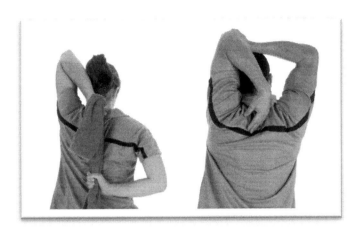

Stretch 1 – Assisted Triceps Stretch:
Stand with one hand behind your neck and your elbow pointing upwards. Then use your other hand (or a rope or towel) to pull your elbow down.

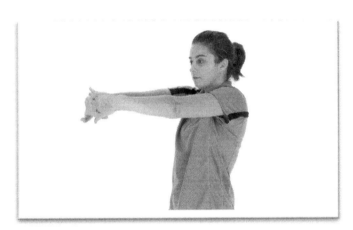

Stretch 2 – Palms-out Forearm Stretch:
Interlock your fingers in front of your chest, then straighten your arms and turn the palms of your hands so that they face outwards.

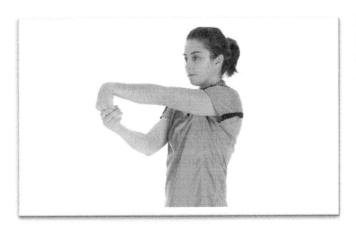

Stretch 3 – Fingers-down Wrist Stretch:
Hold on to your fingers and straighten your arm, then pull your fingers towards your body.

Arms & Hands Stretching Routine #2

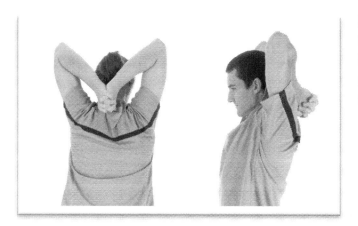

Stretch 1 – Reaching-down Triceps Stretch: Reach behind your head with both hands and your elbows pointing upwards. Then reach down your back with your hands.

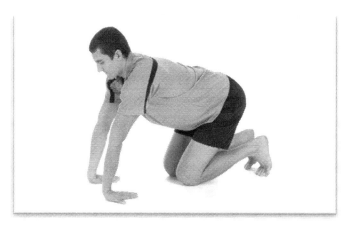

Stretch 2 – Kneeling Forearm Stretch: While crouching on your knees with your forearms facing forward and hands pointing backwards, slowly move rearward.

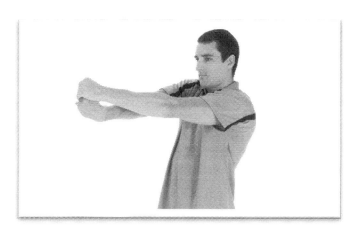

Stretch 3 – Rotating Wrist Stretch: Place one arm straight out in front and parallel to the ground. Rotate your wrist down and outwards and then use your other hand to further rotate your hand upwards.

Arms & Hands Stretching Routine #3

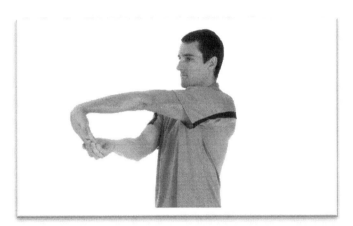

Stretch 1 – Fingers-down Forearm Stretch: Hold onto your fingers and turn your palms outwards. Straighten your arm and then pull your fingers back using your other hand.

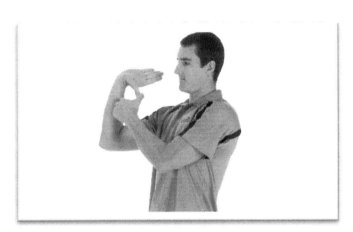

Stretch 2 – Thumb Stretch: Start with your fingers pointing up and your thumb out to one side, then use your other hand to pull your thumb down.

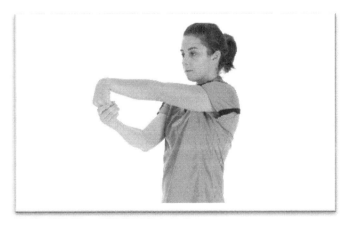

Stretch 3 – Fingers-down Wrist Stretch: Hold on to your fingers and straighten your arm, then pull your fingers towards your body.

Arms & Hands Stretching Routine #4

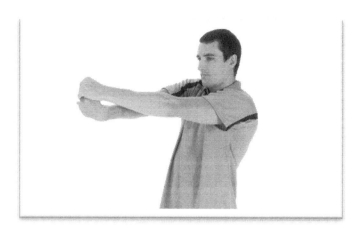

Stretch 1 – Rotating Wrist Stretch: Place one arm straight out in front and parallel to the ground. Rotate your wrist down and outwards and then use your other hand to further rotate your hand upwards.

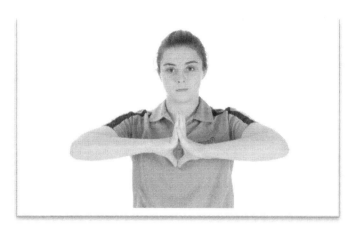

Stretch 2 – Finger Stretch: Place the tips of your fingers together and push your palms towards each other.

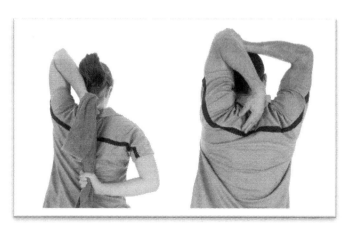

Stretch 3 – Assisted Triceps Stretch: Stand with one hand behind your neck and your elbow pointing upwards. Then use your other hand (or a rope or towel) to pull your elbow down.

Stomach Stretching Routine #1

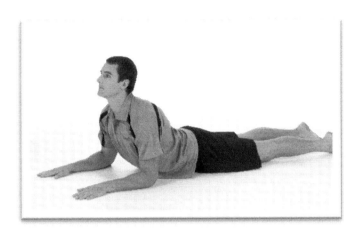

Stretch 1 – On Elbows Stomach Stretch:
Lie face down and bring your hands close to your shoulders. Keep your hips on the ground, look forward and rise up onto your elbows.

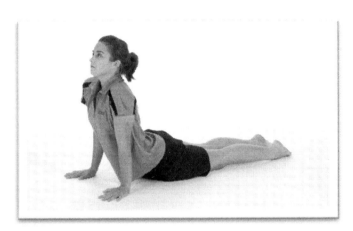

Stretch 2 – Rising Stomach Stretch: Lie face down and bring your hands close to your shoulders. Keep your hips on the ground, look forward and rise up by straightening your arms.

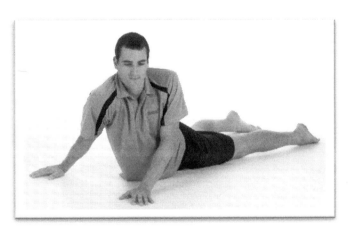

Stretch 3 – Rotating Stomach Stretch: Lie face down and bring your hands close to your shoulders. Keep your hips on the ground, look forward and rise up by straightening your arms. Then slowly bend one arm and rotate that shoulder towards the ground.

Stomach Stretching Routine #2

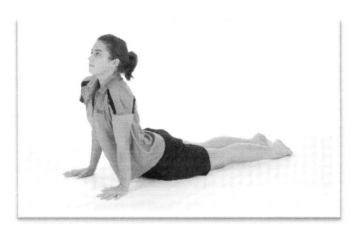

Stretch 1 – Rising Stomach Stretch: Lie face down and bring your hands close to your shoulders. Keep your hips on the ground, look forward and rise up by straightening your arms.

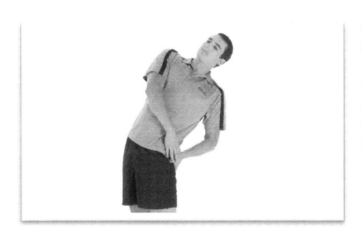

Stretch 2 – Standing Lean-back Side Stomach Stretch: Stand upright with your feet shoulder width apart and place one hand of your buttocks. Look up and slowly lean backwards at the waist, then reach over with your opposite hand and rotate at the waist.

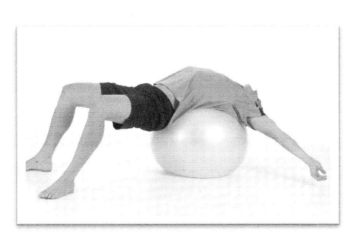

Stretch 3 – Back Arching Stomach Stretch: Sit on a Swiss ball and slowly roll the ball forward while leaning back. Allow your back and shoulders to rest on the ball and your arms to hang to each side.

Stomach Stretching Routine #3

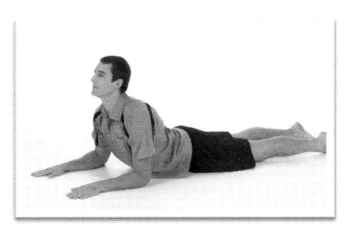

Stretch 1 – On Elbows Stomach Stretch:
Lie face down and bring your hands close to your shoulders. Keep your hips on the ground, look forward and rise up onto your elbows.

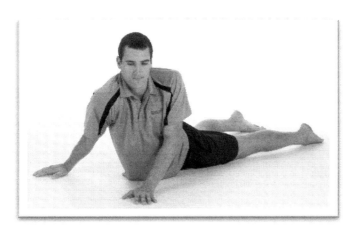

Stretch 2 – Rotating Stomach Stretch:
Lie face down and bring your hands close to your shoulders. Keep your hips on the ground, look forward and rise up by straightening your arms. Then slowly bend one arm and rotate that shoulder towards the ground.

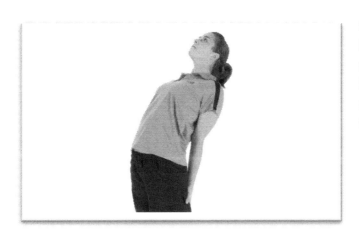

Stretch 3 – Standing Lean-back Stomach Stretch: Stand upright with your feet shoulder width apart and place your hands on your buttocks for support. Look upwards and slowly lean backwards at the waist.

Sides Stretching Routine #1

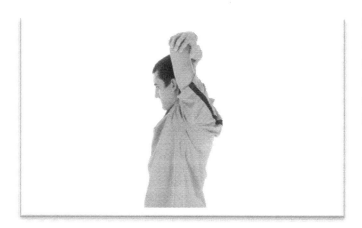

Stretch 1 – Standing Reach-up Back Rotation Stretch: Stand with your feet shoulder width apart. Place your hands above your head while keeping your back and shoulders upright. Slowly rotate your back and shoulders to one side.

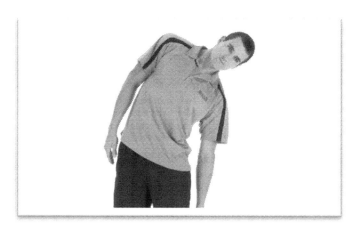

Stretch 2 – Standing Lateral Side Stretch: Stand with your feet about shoulder width apart and look forward. Keep your body upright and slowly bend to the left or right. Reach down your leg with your hand and do not bend forward.

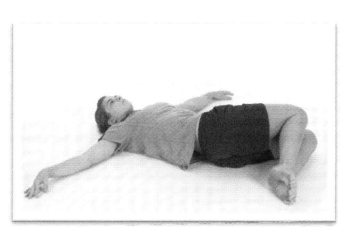

Stretch 3 –Lying Knee Roll-over Stretch: While lying on your back, bend your knees and let them fall to one side. Keep your arms out to the side and let your back and hips rotate with your knees.

Sides Stretching Routine #2

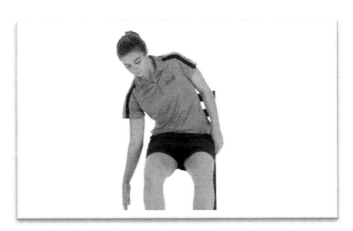

Stretch 1 – Sitting Lateral Side Stretch:
Sit on a chair with your feet flat on the ground, then slowly bend to the left or right while reaching towards the ground. Do not bend forward.

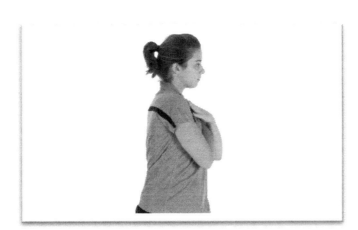

Stretch 2 – Standing Back Rotation Stretch: Stand with your feet shoulder width apart. Place your hands across your chest while keeping your back and shoulders upright. Slowly rotate your shoulders to one side.

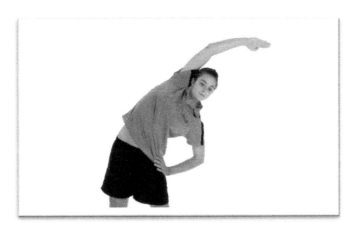

Stretch 3 – Reaching Lateral Side Stretch: Stand with your feet shoulder width apart, then slowly bend to the side and reach over the top of your head with your hand. Do not bend forward.

Upper Back Stretching Routine #1

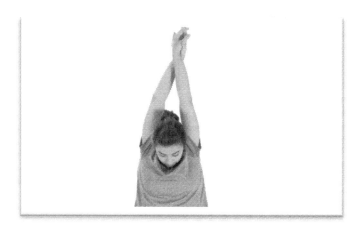

Stretch 1 – Reach-up Back Stretch: Stand with your arms crossed over and then raise them above your head. Let your head fall forward and reach up as high as you can.

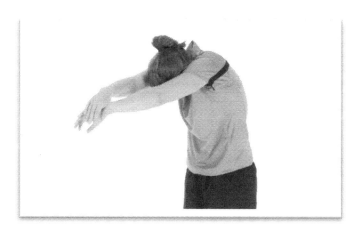

Stretch 2 – Reach Forward Upper Back Stretch: Stand with your arms out in front and your hands crossed over, then push your hands forward as far as possible and let your head fall forward.

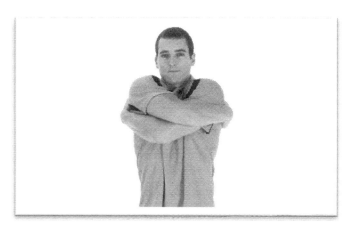

Stretch 3 – Wrap-around Shoulder Stretch: Stand upright and wrap your arms around your shoulders as if hugging yourself. Pull your shoulders back.

Upper Back Stretching Routine #2

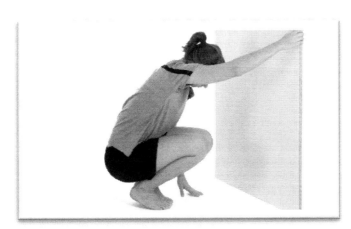

Stretch 1 – Reaching Upper Back Stretch: Sit in a squatting position while facing a door edge or pole, then hold onto the door edge with one hand and lean backwards away from the door.

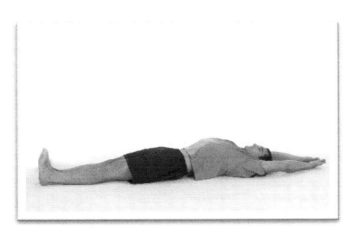

Stretch 2 – Lying Whole Body Stretch: Lie on your back and extend your arms behind you. Keep your toes pointing upwards and lengthen your body as much as you can.

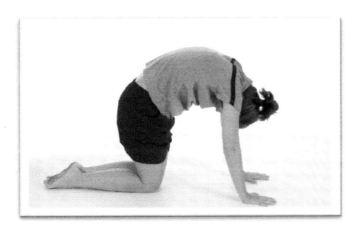

Stretch 3 – Kneeling Back-arch Stretch: Kneel on your hands and knees. Let your head fall forward and arch your back upwards.

Upper Back Stretching Routine #3

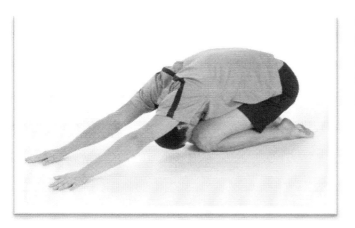

Stretch 1 – Kneeling Reach Forward Stretch: Kneel on the ground and reach forward with your hands. Let your head fall forward and push your buttocks back towards your feet.

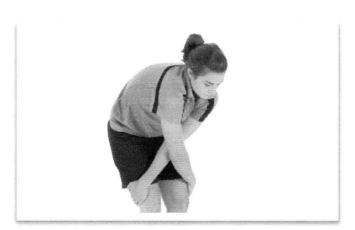

Stretch 2 – Cross-over Shoulder Stretch: Stand with your knees bent. Cross your arms over and grab the back of your knees, then start to rise upwards until you feel tension in your upper back and shoulders.

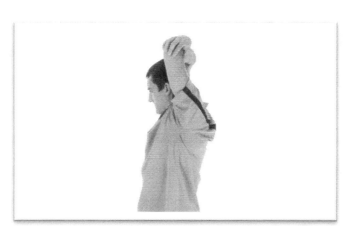

Stretch 3 – Standing Reach-up Back Rotation Stretch: Stand with your feet shoulder width apart. Place your hands above your head while keeping your back and shoulders upright. Slowly rotate your back and shoulders to one side.

Upper Back Stretching Routine #4

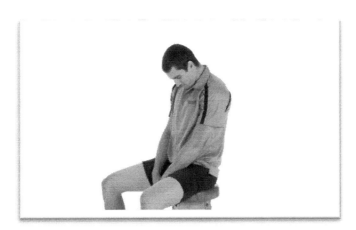

Stretch 1 – Sitting Neck Flexion Stretch: While sitting on a chair, cross your arms and hold onto the chair between your legs. Let your head fall forward and then lean backwards.

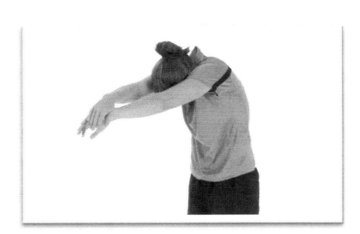

Stretch 2 – Reach Forward Upper Back Stretch: Stand with your arms out in front and your hands crossed over, then push your hands forward as far as possible and let your head fall forward.

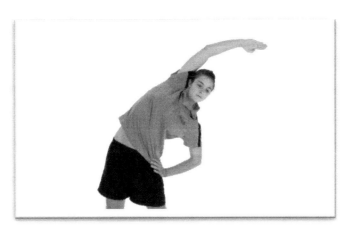

Stretch 3 – Reaching Lateral Side Stretch: Stand with your feet shoulder width apart, then slowly bend to the side and reach over the top of your head with your hand. Do not bend forward.

Lower Back Stretching Routine #1

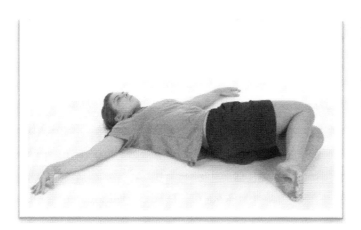

Stretch 1 – Lying Knee Roll-over Stretch: While lying on your back, bend your knees and let them fall to one side. Keep your arms out to the side and let your back and hips rotate with your knees.

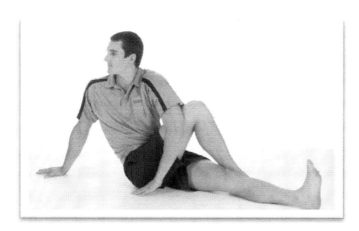

Stretch 2 – Sitting Knee-up Rotation Stretch: Sit with one leg straight and the other leg crossed over your knee. Turn your shoulders and put your arm onto your raised knee to help rotate your shoulders and back.

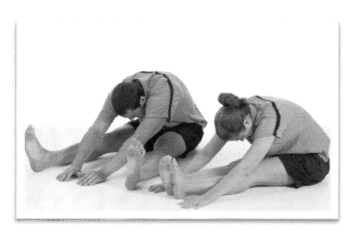

Stretch 3 –Sitting Bent-over Back Stretch: Sit on the ground with your legs straight out in front or at 45 degrees apart. Keep your toes pointing upwards and rest your arms by your side or on your lap. Relax your back and neck and let your head and chest fall forward.

Lower Back Stretching Routine #2

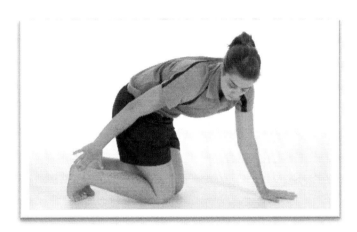

Stretch 1 – Kneeling Reach-around Stretch: Kneel on your hands and knees and then take one hand and reach around towards your ankle. Keep your back parallel to the ground.

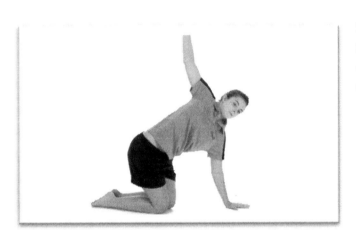

Stretch 2 – Kneeling Back Rotation Stretch: Kneel on the ground and raise one arm upwards while rotating your shoulders and middle back.

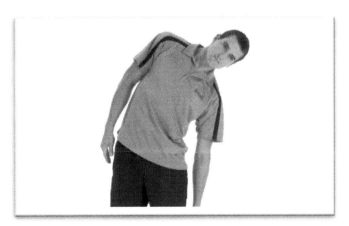

Stretch 3 – Standing Lateral Side Stretch: Stand with your feet about shoulder width apart and look forward. Keep your body upright and slowly bend to the left or right. Reach down your leg with your hand and do not bend forward.

Lower Back Stretching Routine #3

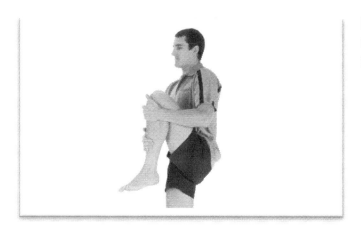

Stretch 1 – Standing Knee-to-chest Stretch: While standing, use your hands to bring one knee into your chest.

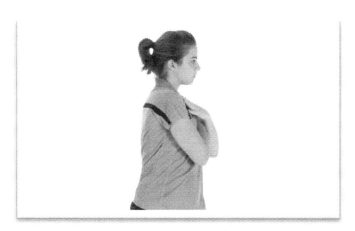

Stretch 2 – Standing Back Rotation Stretch: Stand with your feet shoulder width apart. Place your hands across your chest while keeping your back and shoulders upright. Slowly rotate your shoulders to one side.

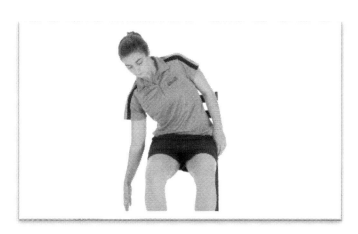

Stretch 3 – Sitting Lateral Side Stretch: Sit on a chair with your feet flat on the ground, then slowly bend to the left or right while reaching towards the ground. Do not bend forward.

Lower Back Stretching Routine #4

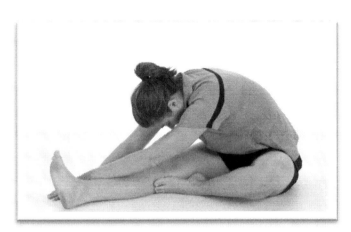

Stretch 1 – Sitting Side Reach Stretch: Sit with one leg straight out to the side and your toes pointing upwards. Then bring your other foot up to your knee and let your head fall forward. Reach towards the outside of your toes with both hands.

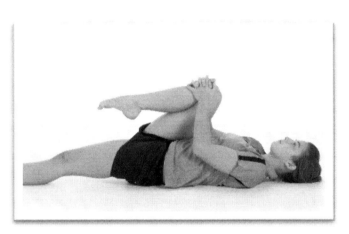

Stretch 2 – Lying Knee-to-chest Stretch: Lie on your back and keep one leg flat on the ground. Use your hands to bring your other knee into your chest.

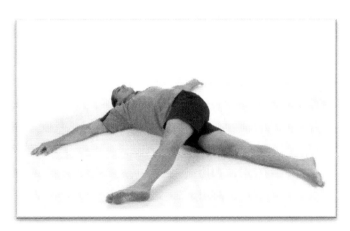

Stretch 3 – Lying Leg Cross-over Stretch: Lie on your back and cross one leg over the other. Keep your arms out to the side and both legs straight. Let your back and hips rotate with your leg.

Lower Back Stretching Routine #5

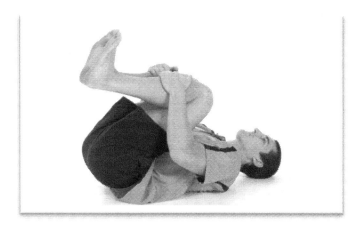

Stretch 1 – Lying Double Knee-to-chest Stretch: Lie on your back and use your hands to bring both knees into your chest.

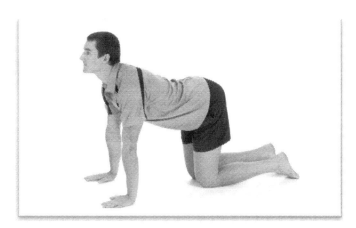

Stretch 2 – Kneeling Back-slump Stretch: Kneel on your hands and knees. Look up and let your back slump downwards.

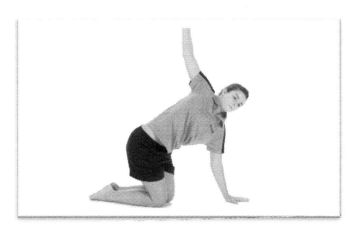

Stretch 3 – Kneeling Back Rotation Stretch: Kneel on the ground and raise one arm upwards while rotating your shoulders and middle back.

Lower Back Stretching Routine #6

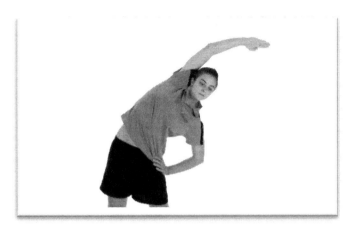

Stretch 1 – Reaching Lateral Side
Stretch: Stand with your feet shoulder width apart, then slowly bend to the side and reach over the top of your head with your hand. Do not bend forward.

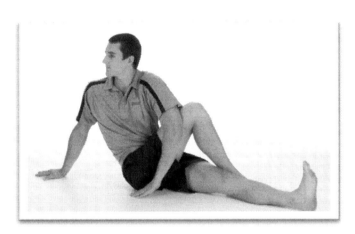

Stretch 2 – Sitting Knee-up Rotation
Stretch: Sit with one leg straight and the other leg crossed over your knee. Turn your shoulders and put your arm onto your raised knee to help rotate your shoulders and back.

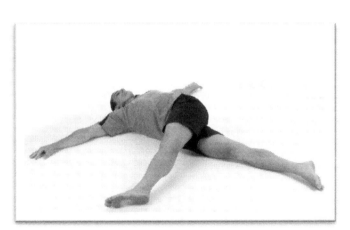

Stretch 3 – Lying Leg Cross-over Stretch:
Lie on your back and cross one leg over the other. Keep your arms out to the side and both legs straight. Let your back and hips rotate with your leg.

Lower Back Stretching Routine #7

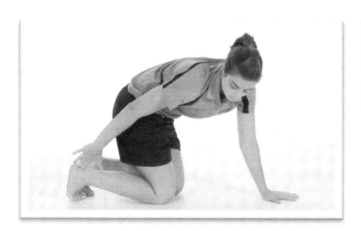

Stretch 1 – Kneeling Reach-around
Stretch: Kneel on your hands and knees and then take one hand and reach around towards your ankle. Keep your back parallel to the ground.

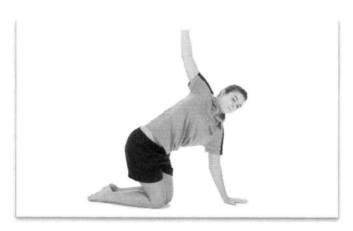

Stretch 2 – Kneeling Back Rotation
Stretch: Kneel on the ground and raise one arm upwards while rotating your shoulders and middle back.

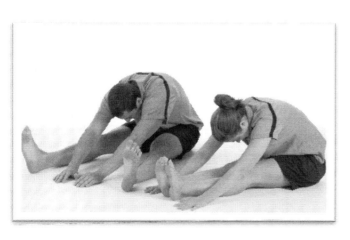

Stretch 3 – Sitting Bent-over Back
Stretch: Sit on the ground with your legs straight out in front or at 45 degrees apart. Keep your toes pointing upwards and rest your arms by your side or on your lap. Relax your back and neck and let your head and chest fall forward.

Lower Back Stretching Routine #8

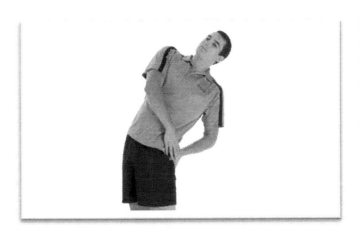

Stretch 1 – Standing Lean-back Side Stomach Stretch: Stand upright with your feet shoulder width apart and place one hand of your buttocks. Look up and slowly lean backwards at the waist, then reach over with your opposite hand and rotate at the waist.

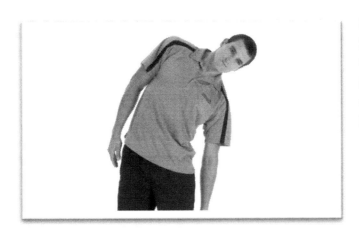

Stretch 2 – Standing Lateral Side Stretch: Stand with your feet about shoulder width apart and look forward. Keep your body upright and slowly bend to the left or right. Reach down your leg with your hand and do not bend forward.

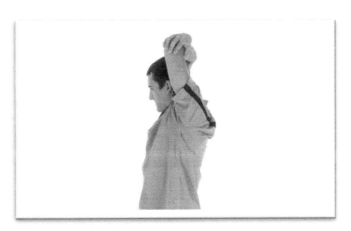

Stretch 3 – Standing Reach-up Back Rotation Stretch: Stand with your feet shoulder width apart. Place your hands above your head while keeping your back and shoulders upright. Slowly rotate your back and shoulders to one side.

Hips Stretching Routine #1

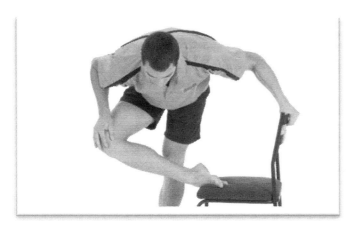

Stretch 1 – Standing Leg Tuck Hip Stretch: Stand beside a chair or table and place the foot furthest from the object onto the object. Relax your leg, lean forward and bend your other leg, lowering yourself towards the ground.

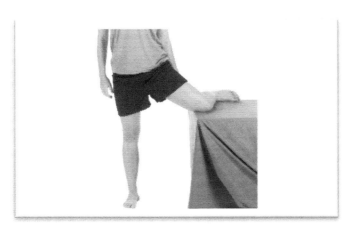

Stretch 2 – Standing Rotational Hip Stretch: Stand beside a table and raise your lower leg out to the side and up onto the table. Then slowly lower your body.

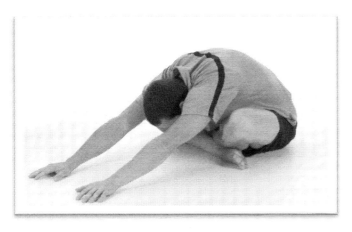

Stretch 3 – Sitting Cross-legged Reach Forward Stretch: Sit with your legs crossed and your knees out, and then gently reach forward.

Hips Stretching Routine #2

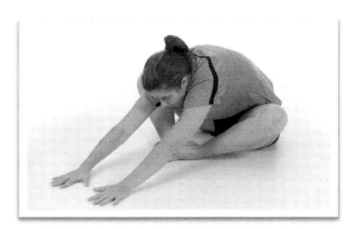

Stretch 1 –Sitting Feet-together Reach Forward Stretch: Sit with the soles of your feet together and your knees out, and then gently reach forward.

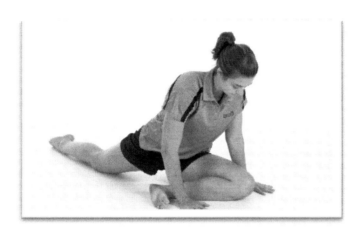

Stretch 2 – Lying Leg Tuck Hip Stretch: Lie face down and bend one leg under your stomach. Lean towards the ground.

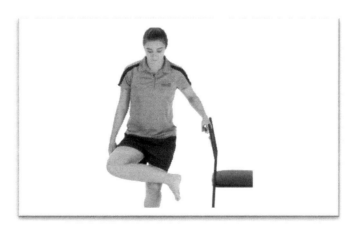

Stretch 3 – Standing Leg Resting Hip Stretch: Stand beside a chair or table for balance, bend one leg and place your other ankle on to your bent knee. Slowly lower yourself towards the ground.

Hips Stretching Routine #3

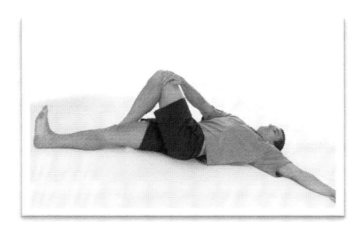

Stretch 1 – Lying Cross-over Knee Pull-down Stretch: Lie on your back and cross one leg over the other. Bring your foot up to your opposite knee and with your opposite arm pull your raised knee down towards the ground.

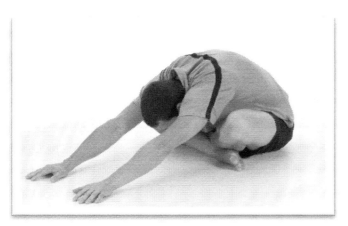

Stretch 2 – Sitting Cross-legged Reach Forward Stretch: Sit with your legs crossed and your knees out, and then gently reach forward.

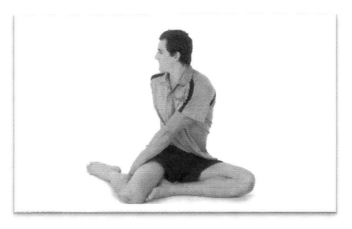

Stretch 3 – Sitting Rotational Hip Stretch: Sit with one leg crossed and your other leg behind your buttocks then lean your whole body towards the leg that is behind your buttocks.

Hips Stretching Routine #4

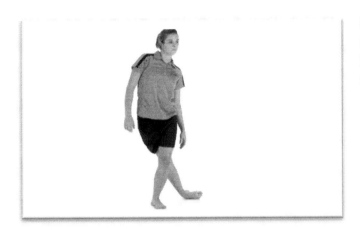

Stretch 1 – Standing Leg-cross Abductor Stretch: Stand upright and cross one foot behind the other. Lean towards the foot that is behind the other.

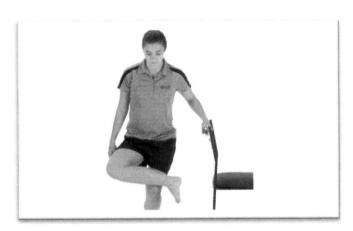

Stretch 2 – Standing Leg Resting Hip Stretch: Stand beside a chair or table for balance, bend one leg and place your other ankle on to your bent knee. Slowly lower yourself towards the ground.

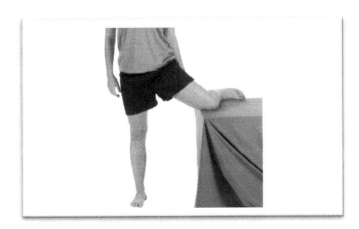

Stretch 3 – Standing Rotational Hip Stretch: Stand beside a table and raise your lower leg out to the side and up onto the table. Then slowly lower your body.

Hips Stretching Routine #5

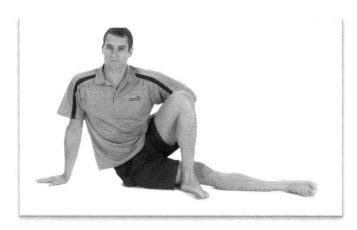

Stretch 1 – Lying Abductor Stretch: Lean on your side on the ground and bring your top leg up to your other knee. Push your body up with your arm and keep your hip on the ground.

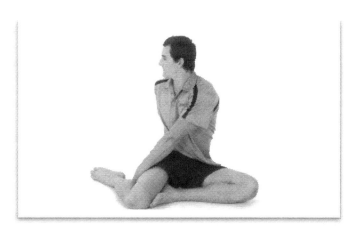

Stretch 2 –Sitting Rotational Hip Stretch: Sit with one leg crossed and your other leg behind your buttocks then lean your whole body towards the leg that is behind your buttocks.

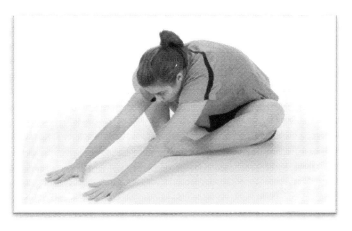

Stretch 3 – Sitting Feet-together Reach Forward Stretch: Sit with the soles of your feet together and your knees out, and then gently reach forward.

Buttocks Stretching Routine #1

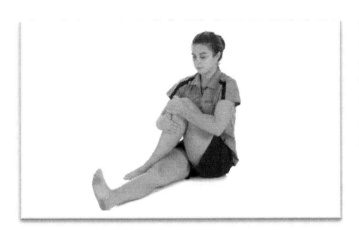

Stretch 1 – Sitting Knee-to-chest Buttocks Stretch: Sit with one leg straight and the other leg crossed over your knee. Pull the raised knee towards your opposite shoulder while keeping your back straight and your shoulders facing forward.

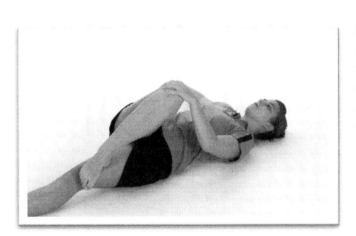

Stretch 2 – Lying Cross-over Knee Pull-up Stretch: Lie on your back and cross one leg over the other. Bring your foot up to your opposite knee and with your opposite arm pull your raised knee up towards your chest.

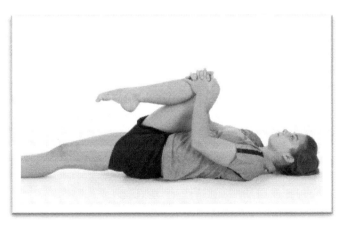

Stretch 3 – Lying Knee-to-chest Stretch: Lie on your back and keep one leg flat on the ground. Use your hands to bring your other knee into your chest.

Buttocks Stretching Routine #2

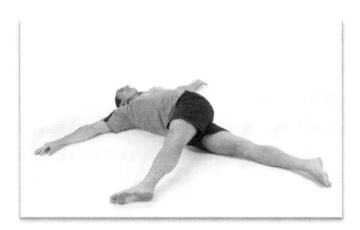

Stretch 1 – Lying Leg Cross-over Stretch: Lie on your back and cross one leg over the other. Keep your arms out to the side and both legs straight. Let your back and hips rotate with your leg.

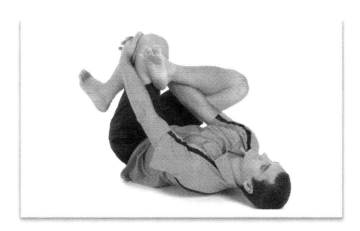

Stretch 2 – Lying Leg Resting Buttocks Stretch: Lie on your back and slightly bend one leg. Raise your other foot up onto your bent leg and rest it on your thigh. Then reach forward, holding onto your knee and pull towards you.

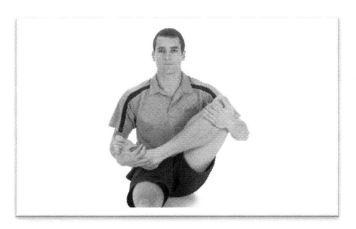

Stretch 3 – Sitting Foot-to-chest Buttocks Stretch: Sit with one leg straight, hold onto your other ankle and then pull it directly towards your chest.

Buttocks Stretching Routine #3

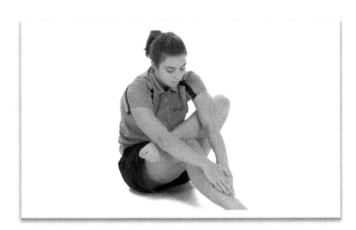

Stretch 1 – Sitting Leg Resting Buttocks Stretch: Sit with one leg slightly bent. Raise your other foot up onto your raised leg and rest it on your thigh, then slowly reach forward.

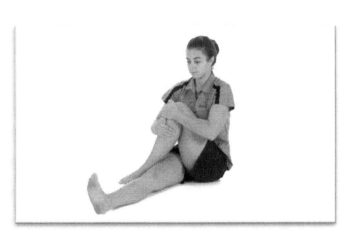

Stretch 2 – Sitting Knee-to-chest Buttocks Stretch: Sit with one leg straight and the other leg crossed over your knee. Pull the raised knee towards your opposite shoulder while keeping your back straight and your shoulders facing forward.

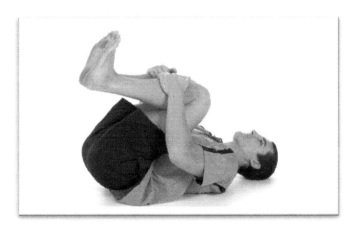

Stretch 3 – Lying Double Knee-to-chest Stretch: Lie on your back and use your hands to bring both knees into your chest.

Buttocks Stretching Routine #4

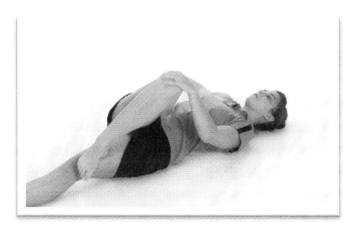

Stretch 1 – Lying Cross-over Knee Pull-up Stretch: Lie on your back and cross one leg over the other. Bring your foot up to your opposite knee and with your opposite arm pull your raised knee up towards your chest.

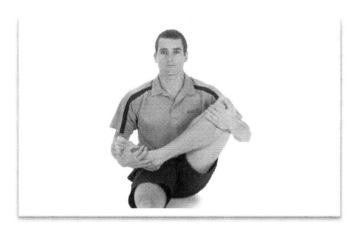

Stretch 2 – Sitting Foot-to-chest Buttocks Stretch: Sit with one leg straight, hold onto your other ankle and then pull it directly towards your chest.

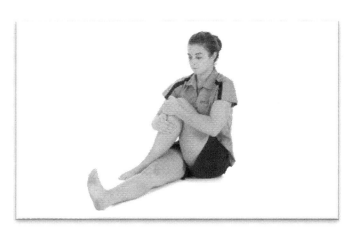

Stretch 3 – Sitting Knee-to-chest Buttocks Stretch: Sit with one leg straight and the other leg crossed over your knee. Pull the raised knee towards your opposite shoulder while keeping your back straight and your shoulders facing forward.

Quadriceps Stretching Routine #1

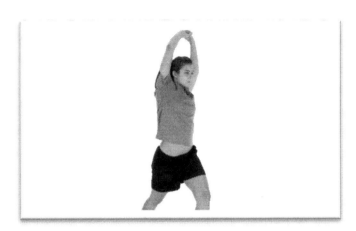

Stretch 1 – Standing Reach-up Quad Stretch: Stand upright and take one small step forward. Reach up with both hands, push your hips forward, lean back and then lean away from your back leg.

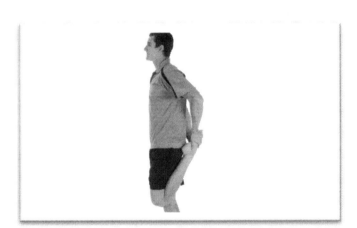

Stretch 2 – Standing Quad Stretch: Stand upright while balancing on one leg. Pull your other foot up behind your buttocks and keep your knees together while pushing your hips forward. Hold on to something for balance if needed.

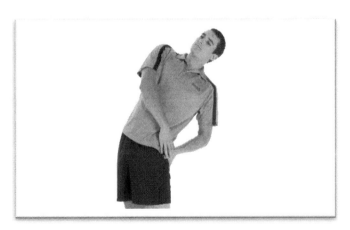

Stretch 3 – Standing Lean-back Side Stomach Stretch: Stand upright with your feet shoulder width apart and place one hand of your buttocks. Look up and slowly lean backwards at the waist, then reach over with your opposite hand and rotate at the waist.

Quadriceps Stretching Routine #2

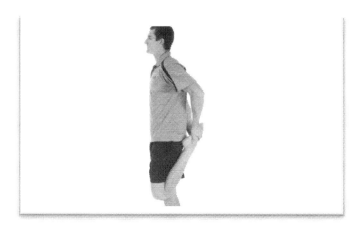

Stretch 1 – Standing Quad Stretch: Stand upright while balancing on one leg. Pull your other foot up behind your buttocks and keep your knees together while pushing your hips forward. Hold on to something for balance if needed.

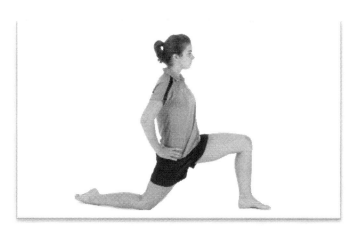

Stretch 2 – Kneeling Quad Stretch: Kneel on one foot and the other knee. If needed, hold on to something to keep your balance and then push your hips forward.

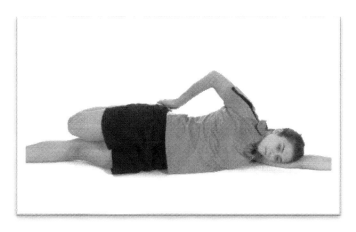

Stretch 3 – Lying Side Quad Stretch: Lie on your side and pull your top leg behind your buttocks. Keep your knees together and push your hips forward.

Quadriceps Stretching Routine #3

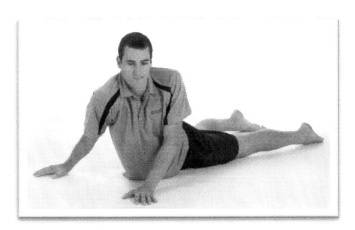

Stretch 1 – Rotating Stomach Stretch:
Lie face down and bring your hands close to your shoulders. Keep your hips on the ground, look forward and rise up by straightening your arms. Then slowly bend one arm and rotate that shoulder towards the ground.

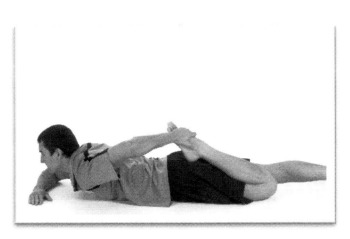

Stretch 2 – Lying Quad Stretch: Lie face down, reach back with one hand and pull one foot up behind your buttocks.

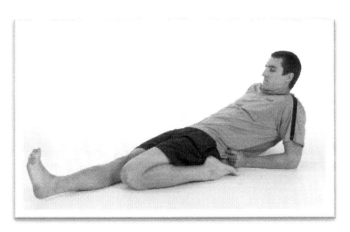

Stretch 3 – Single Lean-back Quad Stretch: Sit on the ground, bend one knee and place that foot next to your buttocks. Then slowly lean backwards.

Quadriceps Stretching Routine #4

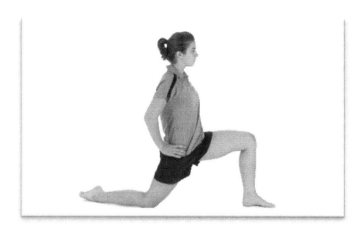

Stretch 1 – Kneeling Quad Stretch: Kneel on one foot and the other knee. If needed, hold on to something to keep your balance and then push your hips forward.

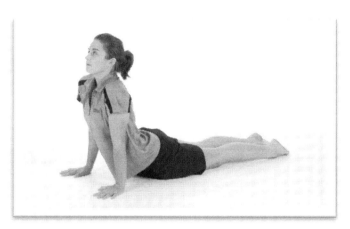

Stretch 2 –Rising Stomach Stretch: Lie face down and bring your hands close to your shoulders. Keep your hips on the ground, look forward and rise up by straightening your arms.

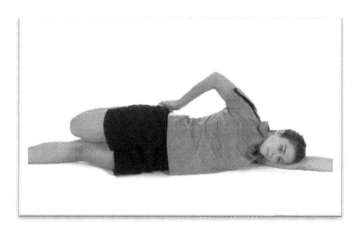

Stretch 3 – Lying Side Quad Stretch: Lie on your side and pull your top leg behind your buttocks. Keep your knees together and push your hips forward.

Hamstrings Stretching Routine #1

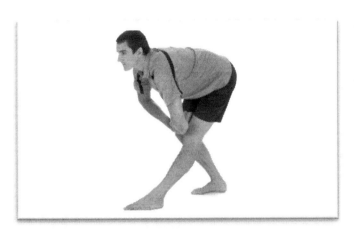

Stretch 1 – Standing Toe-down Hamstring Stretch: Stand with one knee bent and the other leg straight out in front. Point your toes towards the ground and lean forward. Keep your back straight and rest your hands on your bent knee.

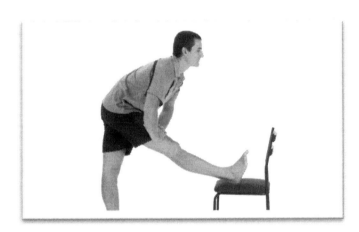

Stretch 2 – Standing Leg-up Hamstring Stretch: Stand upright and raise one leg on to an object. Keep that leg straight and point your toes upwards. Keep your back straight and lean your upper body forward.

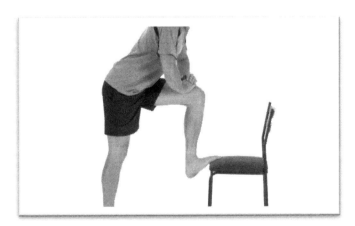

Stretch 3 – Standing Leg-up Bent Knee Hamstring Stretch: Stand with one foot raised onto a chair or an object. Bend your knee and let your heel drop off the edge of the object. Keep your back straight and move your chest towards your raised knee.

Hamstrings Stretching Routine #2

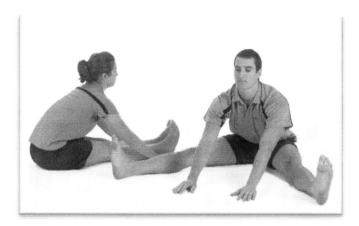

Stretch 1 – Sitting Reach-forward Hamstring Stretch: Sit with both legs straight out in front, or at 45 degrees apart. Keep your toes pointing straight up, make sure your back is straight and then reach forward.

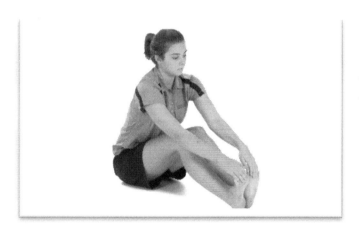

Stretch 2 – Sitting Bent Knee Toe-pull Hamstring Stretch: Sit on the ground with your knees slightly bent. Hold onto your toes with your hands and pull your toes towards your body. Keep your back straight and lean forward.

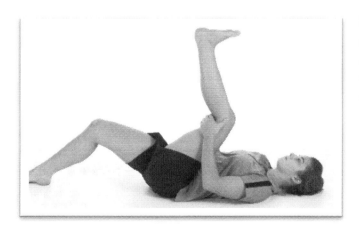

Stretch 3 – Lying Bent Knee Hamstring Stretch: Lie on your back and bend one leg slightly. Pull the other knee towards your chest and then slowly straighten your raised leg.

Hamstrings Stretching Routine #3

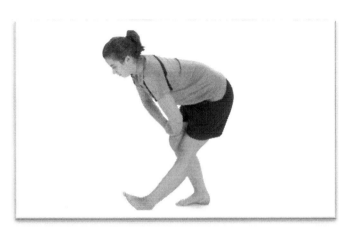

Stretch 1 – Standing Toe-up Hamstring Stretch: Stand with one knee bent and the other leg straight out in front. Point your toes upwards and lean forward. Keep your back straight and rest your hands on your bent knee.

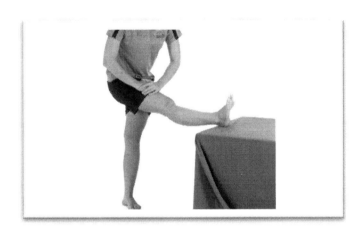

Stretch 2 – Standing Leg-up Toe-in Hamstring Stretch: Stand upright and raise one leg on to an object. Keep that leg straight and point your toes upwards. Then point the toes of your other foot inward and lean forward while keeping your back straight.

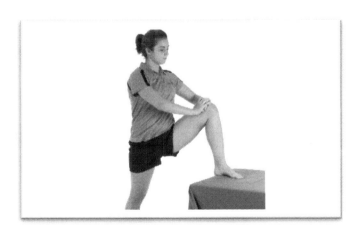

Stretch 3 – Standing Leg-up Toe-in Hamstring Stretch: Stand upright and raise one leg on to an object. Keep that leg straight and point your toes upwards. Then point the toes of your other foot inward and lean forward while keeping your back straight.

Hamstrings Stretching Routine #4

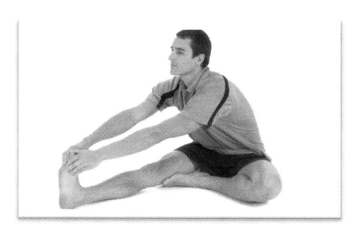

Stretch 1 – Sitting Single Leg Hamstring Stretch: Sit with one leg straight out in front and point your toes upwards. Bring your other foot towards your knee and reach towards your toes with both hands.

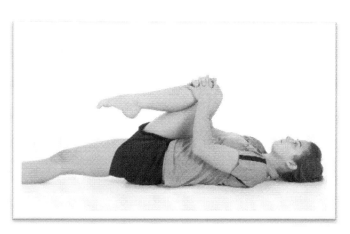

Stretch 2 – Lying Knee-to-chest Stretch: Lie on your back and keep one leg flat on the ground. Use your hands to bring your other knee into your chest.

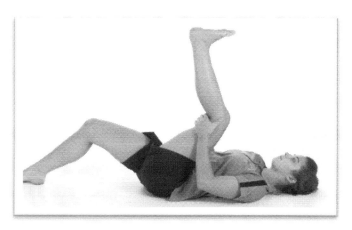

Stretch 3 – Lying Bent Knee Hamstring Stretch: Lie on your back and bend one leg slightly. Pull the other knee towards your chest and then slowly straighten your raised leg.

Hamstrings Stretching Routine #5

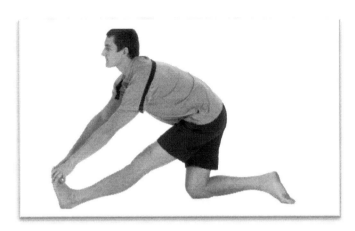

Stretch 1 – Kneeling Toe-up Hamstring Stretch: Kneel on one knee and place your other leg straight forward with your heel on the ground. Keep your back straight and point your toes upwards. Reach towards your toes with one or both hand.

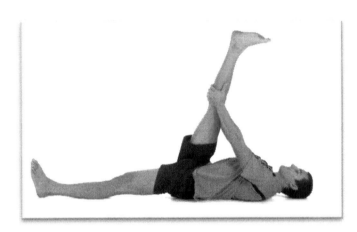

Stretch 2 –Lying Straight Knee Hamstring Stretch: Lie on your back and keep your legs straight. Raise one leg and pull it towards your chest.

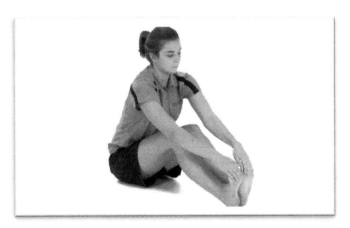

Stretch 3 – Sitting Bent Knee Toe-pull Hamstring Stretch: Sit on the ground with your knees slightly bent. Hold onto your toes with your hands and pull your toes towards your body. Keep your back straight and lean forward.

Hamstrings Stretching Routine #6

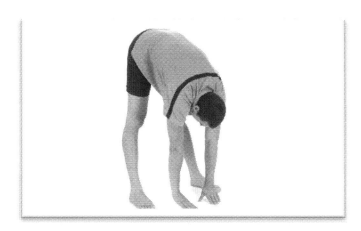

Stretch 1 – Standing Reach-down Hamstring Stretch: Stand with your feet shoulder width apart. Bend forward and reach towards the ground.

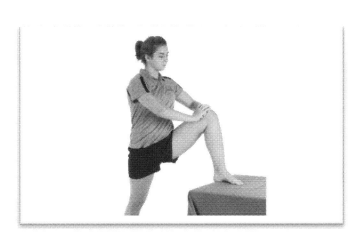

Stretch 2 – Standing High-leg Bent Knee Hamstring Stretch: Stand with one foot raised onto a table. Keep your leg bent and lean your chest into your bent knee.

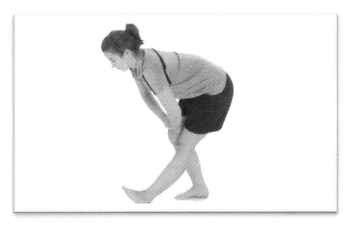

Stretch 3 – Standing Toe-up Hamstring Stretch: Stand with one knee bent and the other leg straight out in front. Point your toes upwards and lean forward. Keep your back straight and rest your hands on your bent knee.

Hamstrings Stretching Routine #7

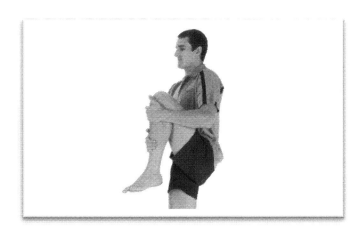

Stretch 1 – Standing Knee-to-chest Stretch: While standing, use your hands to bring one knee into your chest.

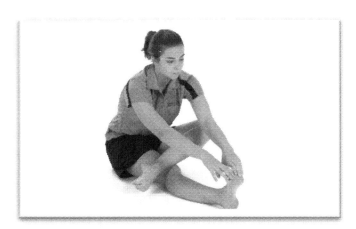

Stretch 2 – Sitting Leg Resting Hamstring Stretch: Sit with one leg straight out in front and your toes pointing upwards. Cross your other leg over and rest your foot on your thigh. Lean forward, keep your back straight and reach for your toes.

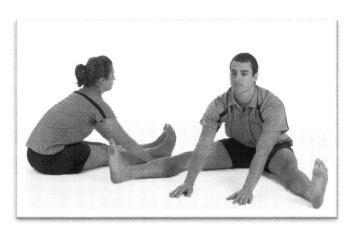

Stretch 3 – Sitting Reach-forward Hamstring Stretch: Sit with both legs straight out in front, or at 45 degrees apart. Keep your toes pointing straight up, make sure your back is straight and then reach forward.

Hamstrings Stretching Routine #8

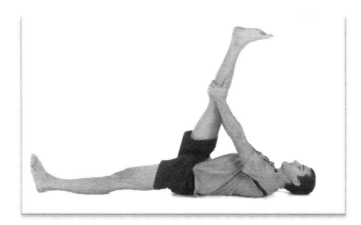

Stretch 1 – Lying Straight Knee Hamstring Stretch: Lie on your back and keep your legs straight. Raise one leg and pull it towards your chest.

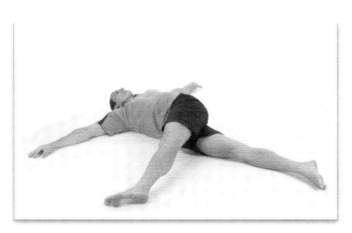

Stretch 2 – Lying Leg Cross-over Stretch: Lie on your back and cross one leg over the other. Keep your arms out to the side and both legs straight. Let your back and hips rotate with your leg.

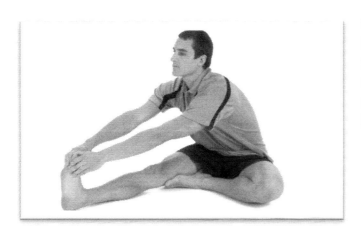

Stretch 3 – Sitting Single Leg Hamstring Stretch: Sit with one leg straight out in front and point your toes upwards. Bring your other foot towards your knee and reach towards your toes with both hands.

Adductors (Groin) Stretching Routine #1

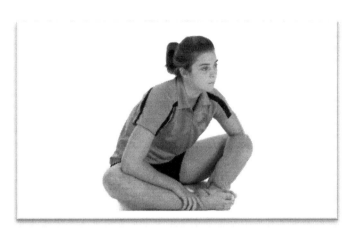

Stretch 1 – Sitting Feet-together Adductor Stretch: Sit with the soles of your feet together and bring your feet towards your groin. Hold onto your ankles and push your knees toward the ground with your elbows. Keep your back straight.

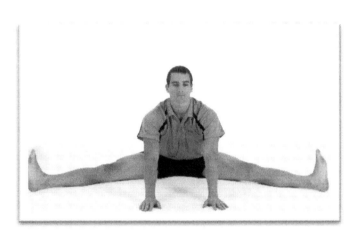

Stretch 2 – Sitting Wide-leg Adductor Stretch: Sit on the ground with your legs straight out and as wide apart as possible and then reach forward while keeping your back straight.

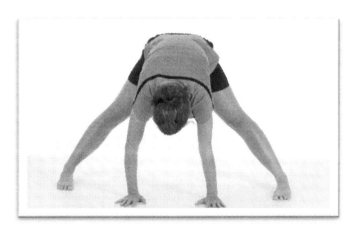

Stretch 3 – Standing Wide-leg Adductor Stretch: Start by standing with your feet wide apart and your toes pointing forward. Then lean forward and reach towards the ground.

Adductors (Groin) Stretching Routine #2

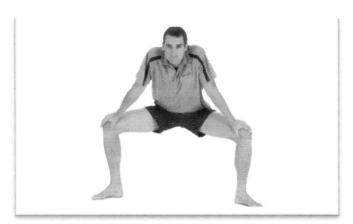

Stretch 1 – Standing Wide Knees Adductor Stretch: Stand with your feet wide apart and your toes pointing diagonally outwards, then bend your knees, lean forward and use your hands to push your knees outwards.

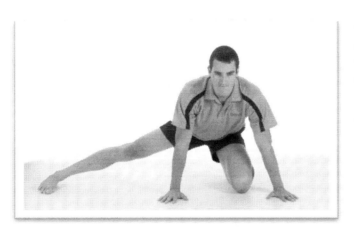

Stretch 2 – Kneeling Leg-out Adductor Stretch: Kneel on one knee and place your other leg out to the side with your toes pointing forward. Rest your hands on the ground and slowly move your foot further out to the side.

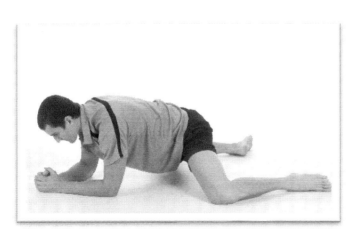

Stretch 3 – Kneeling Face-down Adductor Stretch: Kneel face down with your knees and toes facing out. Lean forward and let your knees move outwards.

Adductors (Groin) Stretching Routine #3

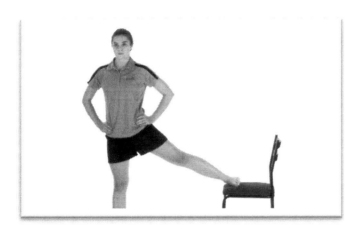

Stretch 1 – Standing Leg-up Adductor Stretch: Stand upright and place one leg out to the side and your foot up on a raised object. Keep your toes facing forward and slowly move your other leg away from the object.

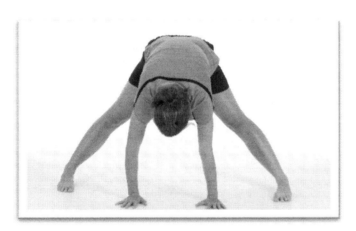

Stretch 2 – Standing Wide-leg Adductor Stretch: Start by standing with your feet wide apart and your toes pointing forward. Then lean forward and reach towards the ground.

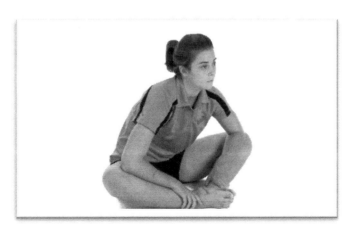

Stretch 3 – Sitting Feet-together Adductor Stretch: Sit with the soles of your feet together and bring your feet towards your groin. Hold onto your ankles and push your knees toward the ground with your elbows. Keep your back straight.

Adductors (Groin) Stretching Routine #4

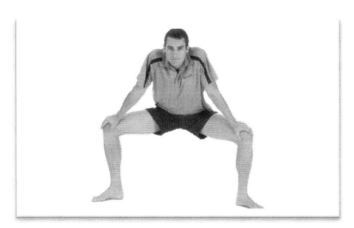

Stretch 1 – Standing Wide Knees Adductor Stretch: Stand with your feet wide apart and your toes pointing diagonally outwards, then bend your knees, lean forward and use your hands to push your knees outwards.

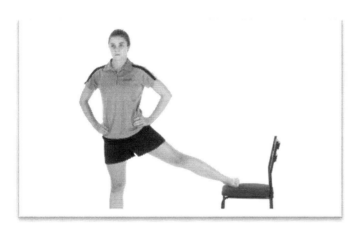

Stretch 2 –Standing Leg-up Adductor Stretch: Stand upright and place one leg out to the side and your foot up on a raised object. Keep your toes facing forward and slowly move your other leg away from the object.

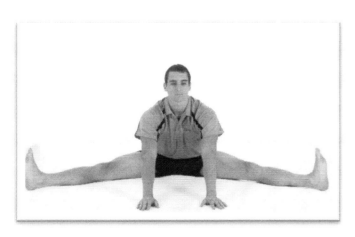

Stretch 3 – Sitting Wide-leg Adductor Stretch: Sit on the ground with your legs straight out and as wide apart as possible and then reach forward while keeping your back straight.

Adductors (Groin) Stretching Routine #5

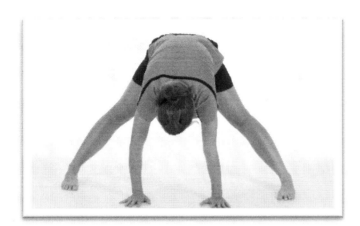

Stretch 1 – Standing Wide-leg Adductor Stretch: Start by standing with your feet wide apart and your toes pointing forward. Then lean forward and reach towards the ground.

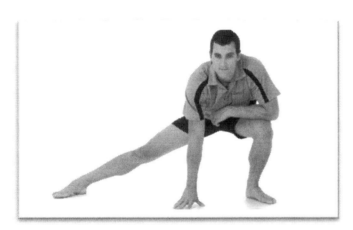

Stretch 2 – Squatting Leg-out Adductor Stretch: Stand with your feet wide apart. Keep one leg straight and your toes pointing forward while bending the other leg and turning your toes out to the side. Lower your groin towards the ground and rest your hands on your bent knee or the ground.

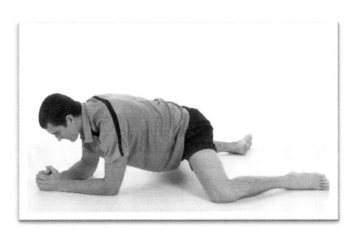

Stretch 3 – Kneeling Face-down Adductor Stretch: Kneel face down with your knees and toes facing out. Lean forward and let your knees move outwards.

Abductors Stretching Routine #1

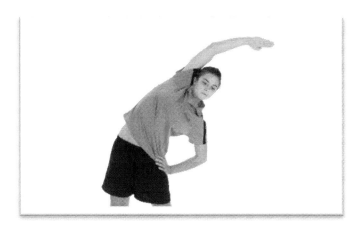

Stretch 1 – Reaching Lateral Side Stretch:
Stand with your feet shoulder width apart, then slowly bend to the side and reach over the top of your head with your hand. Do not bend forward.

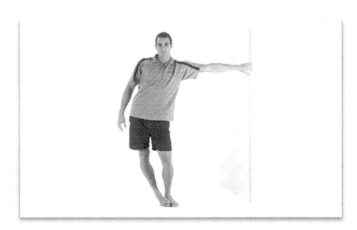

Stretch 2 – Leaning Abductor Stretch:
While standing next to a pole, or door jam, hold onto the pole with one hand. Keep your feet together, and lean your hips away from the pole. Keep your outside leg straight and bend your inside leg slightly.

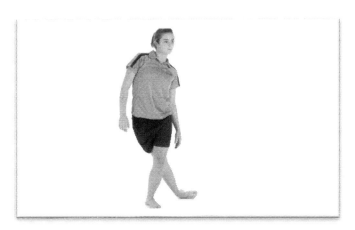

Stretch 3 – Standing Leg-cross Abductor Stretch:
Stand upright and cross one foot behind the other. Lean towards the foot that is behind the other.

Abductors Stretching Routine #2

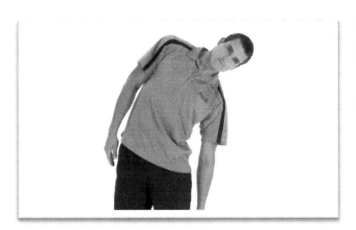

Stretch 1 – Standing Lateral Side Stretch: Stand with your feet about shoulder width apart and look forward. Keep your body upright and slowly bend to the left or right. Reach down your leg with your hand and do not bend forward.

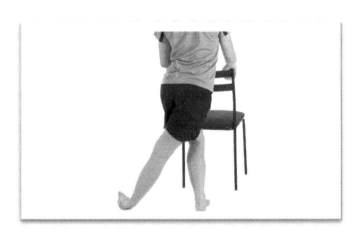

Stretch 2 – Standing Leg-under Abductor Stretch: While standing lean forward and hold onto a chair or bench to help with balance. Cross one foot behind the other and slide that foot to the side. Keep your leg straight and slowly bend your front leg to lower your body.

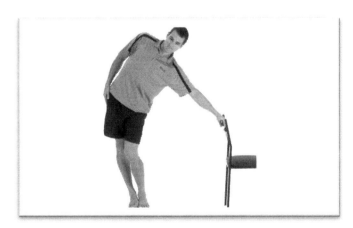

Stretch 3 – Standing Hip-out Abductor Stretch: Stand upright beside a chair or table with both feet together. Lean your upper body towards the chair while pushing your hips away from the chair. Keep your outside leg straight and bend your inside leg slightly.

Abductors Stretching Routine #3

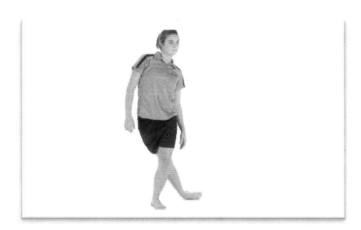

Stretch 1 – Standing Leg-cross Abductor Stretch: Stand upright and cross one foot behind the other. Lean towards the foot that is behind the other.

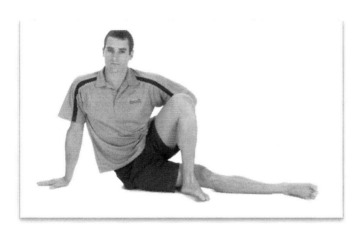

Stretch 2 – Lying Abductor Stretch: Lean on your side on the ground and bring your top leg up to your other knee. Push your body up with your arm and keep your hip on the ground.

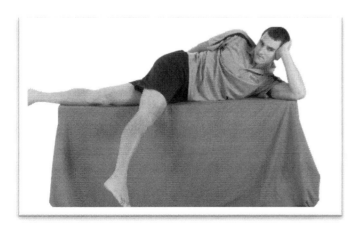

Stretch 3 – Lying Leg-hang Abductor Stretch: Lie on your side on a bench, let your top leg fall forward and off the side of the bench.

Upper Calves Stretching Routine #1

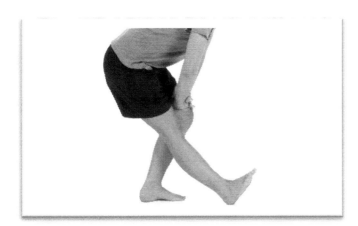

Stretch 1 – Standing Toe Raised Calf Stretch: Stand with one knee bent and the other leg straight out in front. Point your toes upwards and lean forward. Keep your back straight and rest your hands on your bent knee.

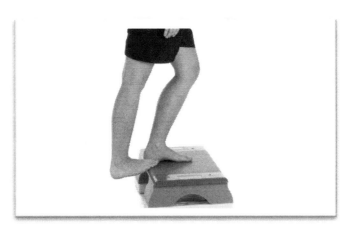

Stretch 2 – Single Heel-drop Calf Stretch: Stand on a raised object or step. Put the ball of one foot on the edge of the step and keep your leg straight. Let your heel drop towards the ground.

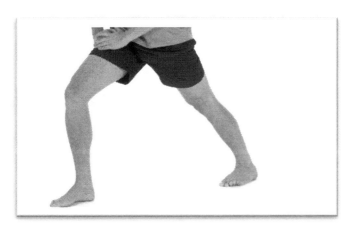

Stretch 3 – Standing Heel-back Calf Stretch: Stand upright and take one big step backwards. Keep your back leg straight, your toes pointing forward and push your heel to the ground.

Upper Calves Stretching Routine #2

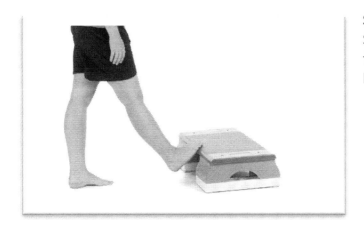

Stretch 1 – Standing Toe-up Calf Stretch: Stand upright and place the ball of your foot on a step or raised object. Keep your leg straight and lean towards your toes.

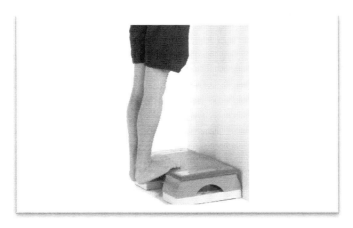

Stretch 2 – Double Heel-drop Calf Stretch: Stand on a raised object or step. Put the balls of both feet on the edge of the step and keep your legs straight. Let your heels drop towards the ground.

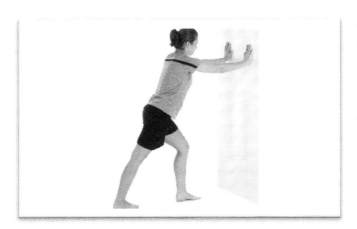

Stretch 3 – Leaning Heel-back Calf Stretch: Reach towards a wall and place one foot as far from the wall as is comfortable. Make sure that both toes are pointing forward and your heel is on the ground. Keep your back leg straight and lean towards the wall.

Upper Calves Stretching Routine #3

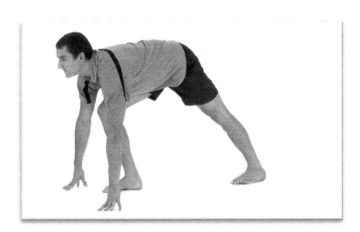

Stretch 1 – Crouching Heel-back Calf Stretch: Stand upright and place one foot in front of the other. Bend your front leg and keep your back leg straight. Push your heel to the ground and lean forward. Place your hands on the ground in front of you.

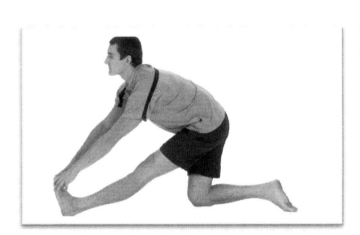

Stretch 2 –Kneeling Toe-up Calf Stretch: Kneel on one knee and place your other leg straight forward with your heel on the ground. Keep your back straight and point your toes upwards. Reach towards your toes with one or both hand.

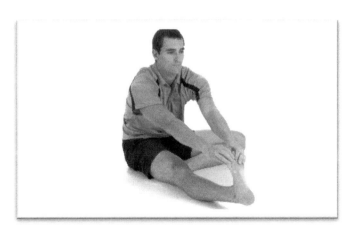

Stretch 3 – Sitting Toe-pull Calf Stretch: Sit with one leg straight out in front and your toes pointing upwards. Reach forward and pull your toes back towards your body.

Upper Calves Stretching Routine #4

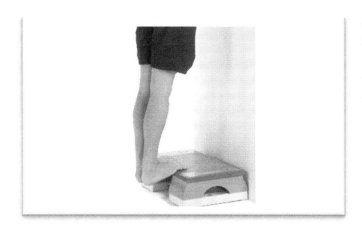

Stretch 1 – Double Heel-drop Calf Stretch: Stand on a raised object or step. Put the balls of both feet on the edge of the step and keep your legs straight. Let your heels drop towards the ground.

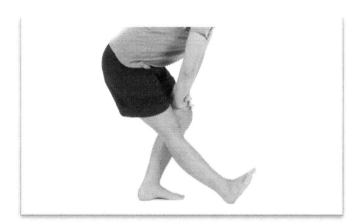

Stretch 2 – Standing Toe Raised Calf Stretch: Stand with one knee bent and the other leg straight out in front. Point your toes upwards and lean forward. Keep your back straight and rest your hands on your bent knee.

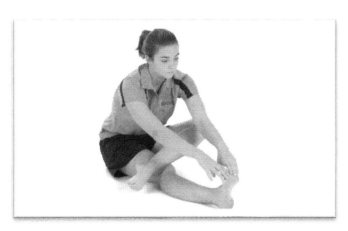

Stretch 3 – Sitting Leg Resting Calf Stretch: Sit with one leg straight out in front and your toes pointing upwards. Cross your other leg over and rest your foot on your thigh. Lean forward, keep your back straight and reach for your toes.

Lower Calves & Achilles Stretching Routine #1

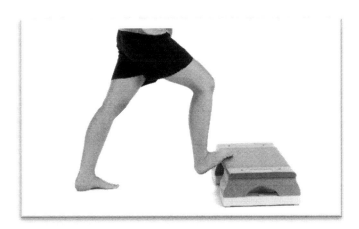

Stretch 1 – Standing Toe-up Achilles Stretch: Stand upright and place the ball of your foot onto a step or raised object. Bend your knee and lean forward.

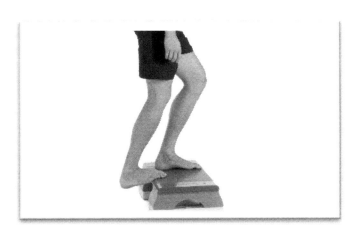

Stretch 2 – Single Heel-drop Achilles Stretch: Stand on a raised object or step and place the ball of one of your feet on the edge of the step. Bend your knee slightly and let your heel drop towards the ground.

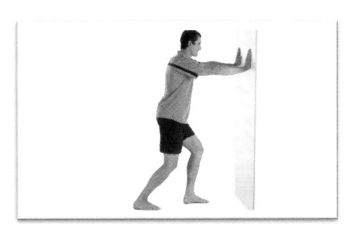

Stretch 3 – Leaning Heel-back Achilles Stretch: Reach towards a wall and place one foot as far from the wall as is comfortable. Make sure that both toes are pointing forward and your heels are on the ground. Bend your back knee and lean towards the wall.

Lower Calves & Achilles Stretching Routine #2

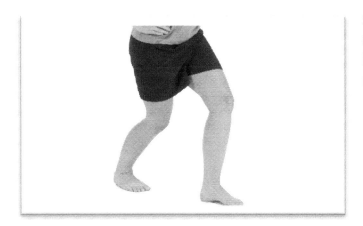

Stretch 1 – Standing Heel-back Achilles Stretch: Stand upright and take one step backwards. Bend your back knee and push your heel towards the ground.

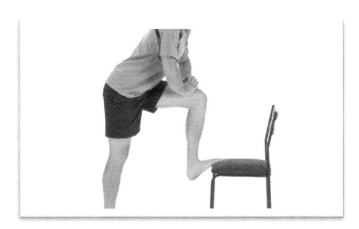

Stretch 2 – Standing Leg-up Bent Knee Achilles Stretch: Stand with one foot raised onto a chair or an object. Bend your knee and let your heel drop off the edge of the object. Keep your back straight, move your chest towards your raised knee and push your heel towards the ground.

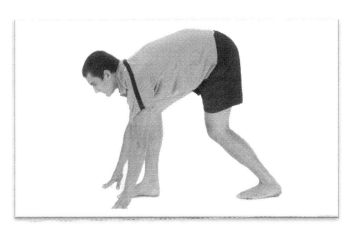

Stretch 3 – Crouching Heel-back Achilles Stretch: Stand upright and place one foot in front of the other. Bend your front leg and your back leg and then push your back heel towards the ground. Lean forward and place your hands on the ground in front of you.

Lower Calves & Achilles Stretching Routine #3

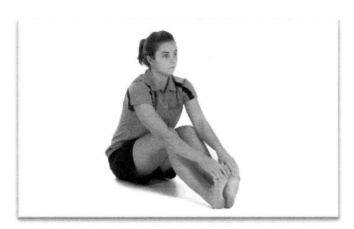

Stretch 1 – Sitting Toe-pull Achilles Stretch: Sit on the ground with your knees slightly bent. Hold onto your toes with your hands and pull your toes towards your body.

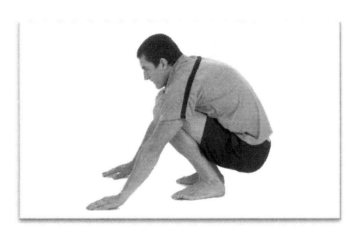

Stretch 2 – Squatting Achilles Stretch: Stand with your feet shoulder width apart. Then bend your legs and lower your body into a sitting position. Place your hands out in front for balance.

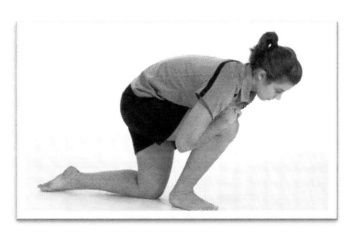

Stretch 3 – Kneeling Heel-down Achilles Stretch: Kneel on one foot and place your body weight over your knee. Keep your heel on the ground and lean forward.

Lower Calves & Achilles Stretching Routine #4

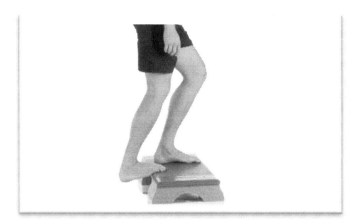

Stretch 1 – Single Heel-drop Achilles Stretch: Stand on a raised object or step and place the ball of one of your feet on the edge of the step. Bend your knee slightly and let your heel drop towards the ground.

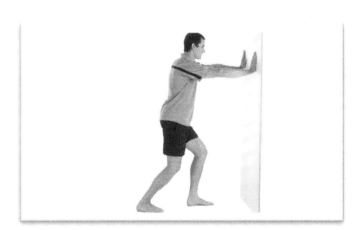

Stretch 2 – Leaning Heel-back Achilles Stretch: Reach towards a wall and place one foot as far from the wall as is comfortable. Make sure that both toes are pointing forward and your heels are on the ground. Bend your back knee and lean towards the wall.

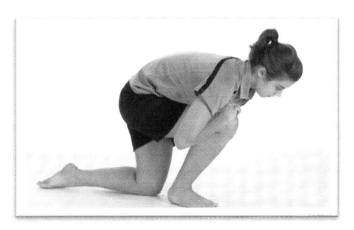

Stretch 3 – Kneeling Heel-down Achilles Stretch: Kneel on one foot and place your body weight over your knee. Keep your heel on the ground and lean forward.

Shins, Ankles, Feet & Toes
Stretching Routine #1

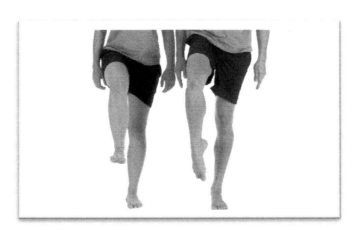

Stretch 1 – Ankle Rotation Stretch: Raise one foot off the ground and slowly rotate your foot and ankle in all directions.

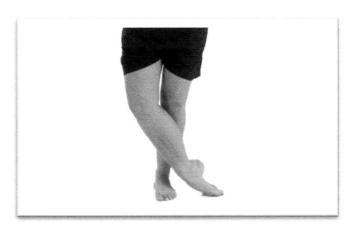

Stretch 2 – Front Cross-over Shin Stretch: Stand upright and place the top of your toes on the ground in front of your other foot. Slowly bend your other knee to force your ankle to the ground.

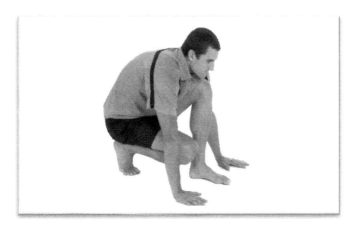

Stretch 3 – Squatting Toe Stretch: Kneel on one foot with your hands on the ground. Keep the toes of your rear foot on the ground, slowly lean forward and arch your foot.

Shins, Ankles, Feet & Toes
Stretching Routine #2

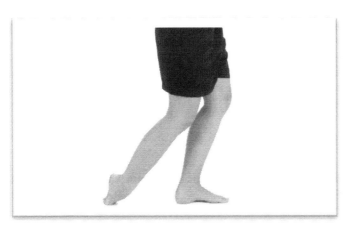

Stretch 1 – Foot-behind Shin Stretch:
Stand upright and place the top of your toes on the ground behind you. Push your ankle to the ground.

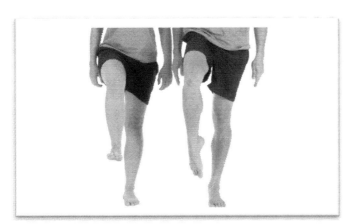

Stretch 2 – Ankle Rotation Stretch: Raise one foot off the ground and slowly rotate your foot and ankle in all directions.

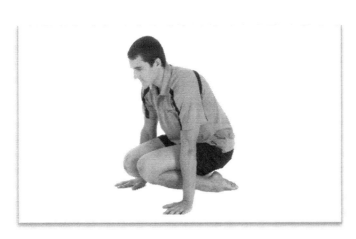

Stretch 3 – Double Kneeling Shin Stretch: Sit with your knees and feet flat on the ground. Sit back on your ankles and keep your knees together. Place your hands next to your knees and slowly lean backwards while raising your knees off the ground.

Stretching Routines for Injuries

Stretching Routine for
Whiplash & Wryneck #1

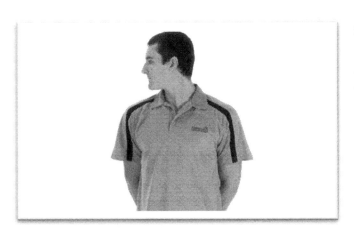

Stretch 1 – Rotating Neck Stretch: Stand upright while keeping your shoulders still and your head up, then slowly rotate your chin towards your shoulder.

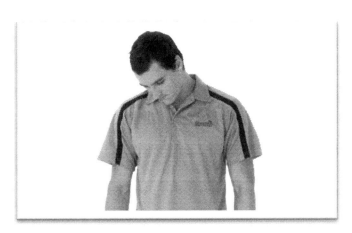

Stretch 2 – Diagonal Flexion Neck Stretch: Stand upright and let your chin fall forward towards your chest. Then gently lean your head to one side.

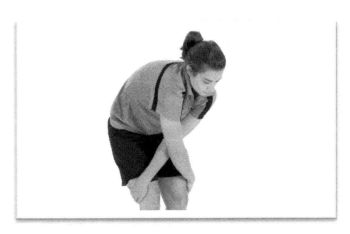

Stretch 3 – Cross-over Shoulder Stretch: Stand with your knees bent. Cross your arms over and grab the back of your knees, then start to rise upwards until you feel tension in your upper back and shoulders.

Stretching Routine for Whiplash & Wryneck #2

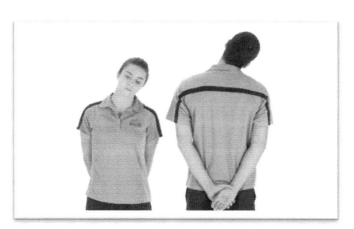

Stretch 1 – Lateral Neck Stretch: Look forward while keeping your head up. Slowly move your ear towards your shoulder while keeping your hands behind your back.

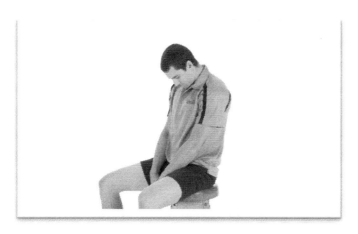

Stretch 2 – Sitting Neck Flexion Stretch: While sitting on a chair, cross your arms and hold onto the chair between your legs. Let your head fall forward and then lean backwards.

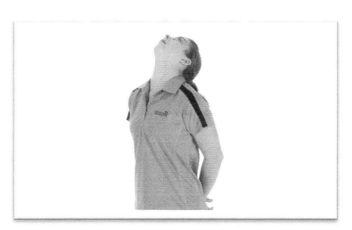

Stretch 3 – Neck Extension Stretch: Stand upright and lift your head, looking upwards as if trying to point up with your chin. Relax your shoulders and keep your hands by your side.

Stretching Routine for Thumb Sprain #1

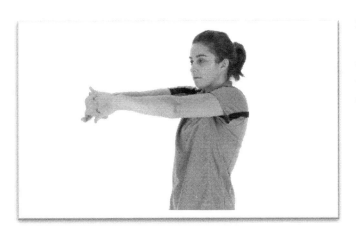

Stretch 1 – Palms-out Forearm Stretch: Interlock your fingers in front of your chest, then straighten your arms and turn the palms of your hands so that they face outwards.

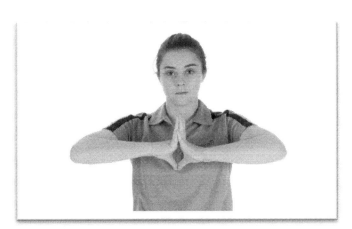

Stretch 2 – Finger Stretch: Place the tips of your fingers together and push your palms towards each other.

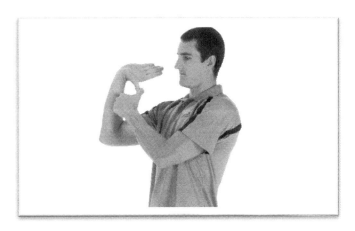

Stretch 3 – Thumb Stretch: Start with your fingers pointing up and your thumb out to one side, then use your other hand to pull your thumb down.

Stretching Routine for
Thumb Sprain #2

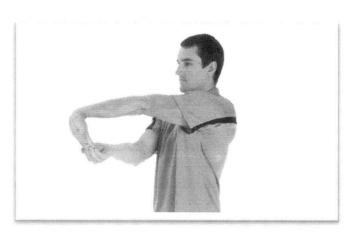

Stretch 1 – Fingers-down Forearm Stretch: Hold onto your fingers and turn your palms outwards. Straighten your arm and then pull your fingers back using your other hand.

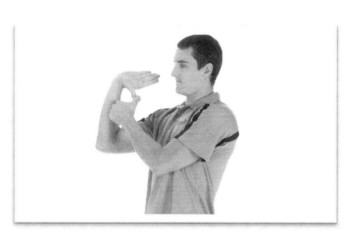

Stretch 2 – Thumb Stretch: Start with your fingers pointing up and your thumb out to one side, then use your other hand to pull your thumb down.

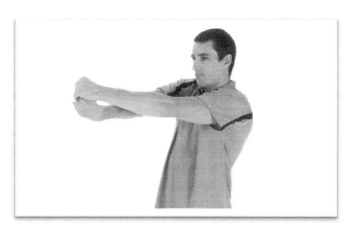

Stretch 3 – Rotating Wrist Stretch: Place one arm straight out in front and parallel to the ground. Rotate your wrist down and outwards and then use your other hand to further rotate your hand upwards.

Stretching Routine for
Finger Sprain & Tendinitis #1

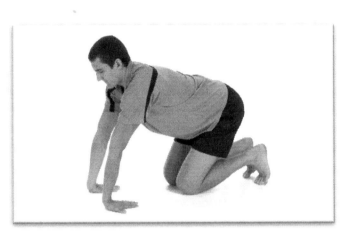

Stretch 1 – Kneeling Forearm Stretch: While crouching on your knees with your forearms facing forward and hands pointing backwards, slowly move rearward.

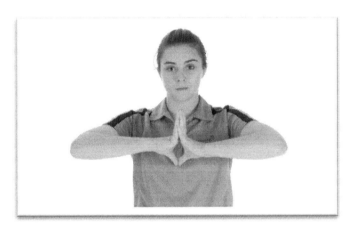

Stretch 2 – Finger Stretch: Place the tips of your fingers together and push your palms towards each other.

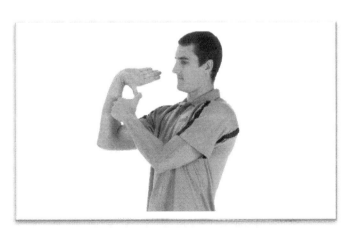

Stretch 3 – Thumb Stretch: Start with your fingers pointing up and your thumb out to one side, then use your other hand to pull your thumb down.

Stretching Routine for
Finger Sprain & Tendinitis #2

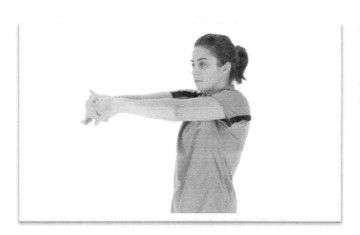

Stretch 1 – Palms-out Forearm Stretch: Interlock your fingers in front of your chest, then straighten your arms and turn the palms of your hands so that they face outwards.

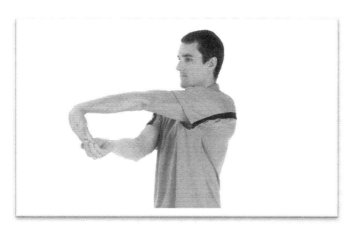

Stretch 2 – Fingers-down Forearm Stretch: Hold onto your fingers and turn your palms outwards. Straighten your arm and then pull your fingers back using your other hand.

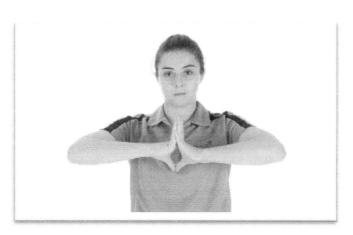

Stretch 3 – Finger Stretch: Place the tips of your fingers together and push your palms towards each other.

Stretching Routine for
Wrist Sprain & Tendinitis #1

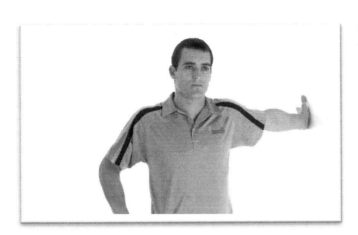

Stretch 1 – Forearm Stretch: Stand with your arm extended to the rear and parallel to the ground. Hold on to an immovable object and then turn your shoulders and body away from your outstretched arm.

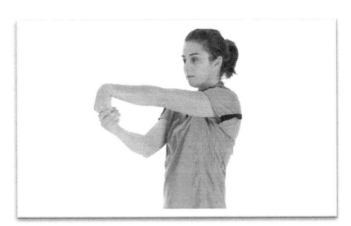

Stretch 2 – Fingers-down Wrist Stretch: Hold on to your fingers and straighten your arm, then pull your fingers towards your body.

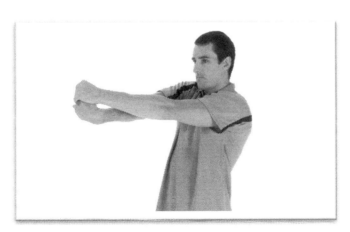

Stretch 3 – Rotating Wrist Stretch: Place one arm straight out in front and parallel to the ground. Rotate your wrist down and outwards and then use your other hand to further rotate your hand upwards.

Stretching Routine for Wrist Sprain & Tendinitis #2

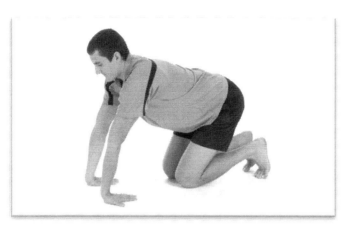

Stretch 1 – Kneeling Forearm Stretch:
While crouching on your knees with your forearms facing forward and hands pointing backwards, slowly move rearward.

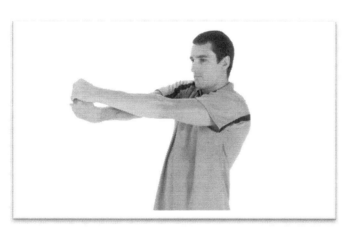

Stretch 2 – Rotating Wrist Stretch: Place one arm straight out in front and parallel to the ground. Rotate your wrist down and outwards and then use your other hand to further rotate your hand upwards.

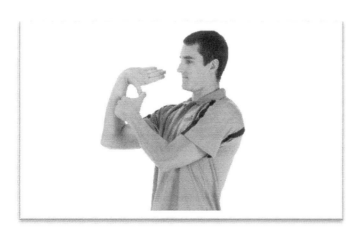

Stretch 3 – Thumb Stretch: Start with your fingers pointing up and your thumb out to one side, then use your other hand to pull your thumb down.

Stretching Routine for
Carpel Tunnel & Ulnar Tunnel Syndrome #1

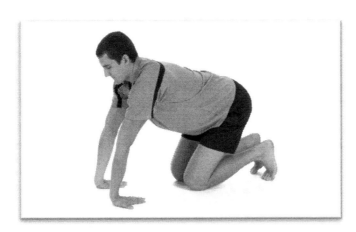

Stretch 1 – Kneeling Forearm Stretch:
While crouching on your knees with your forearms facing forward and hands pointing backwards, slowly move rearward.

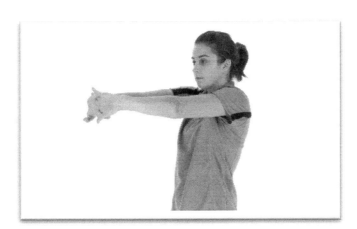

Stretch 2 – Palms-out Forearm Stretch:
Interlock your fingers in front of your chest, then straighten your arms and turn the palms of your hands so that they face outwards.

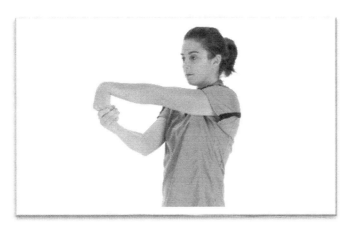

Stretch 3 – Fingers-down Wrist Stretch:
Hold on to your fingers and straighten your arm, then pull your fingers towards your body.

Stretching Routine for
Carpel Tunnel & Ulnar Tunnel Syndrome #2

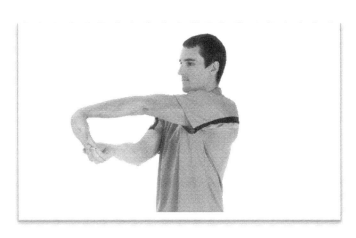

Stretch 1 – Fingers-down Forearm Stretch: Hold onto your fingers and turn your palms outwards. Straighten your arm and then pull your fingers back using your other hand.

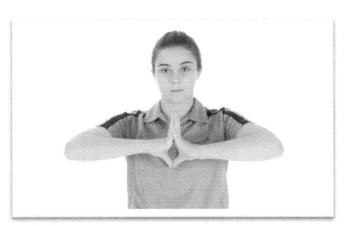

Stretch 2 – Finger Stretch: Place the tips of your fingers together and push your palms towards each other.

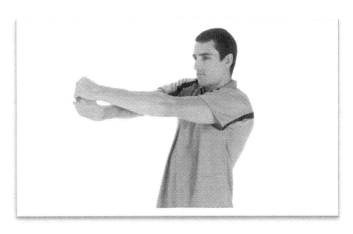

Stretch 3 – Rotating Wrist Stretch: Place one arm straight out in front and parallel to the ground. Rotate your wrist down and outwards and then use your other hand to further rotate your hand upwards.

Stretching Routine for
Elbow Sprain #1

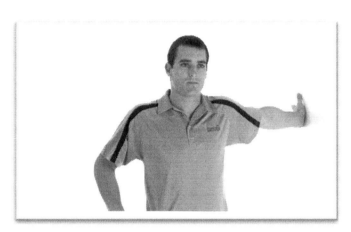

Stretch 1 – Parallel Arm Forearm
Stretch: Stand with your arm extended to the rear and parallel to the ground. Hold on to an immovable object and then turn your shoulders and body away from your outstretched arm.

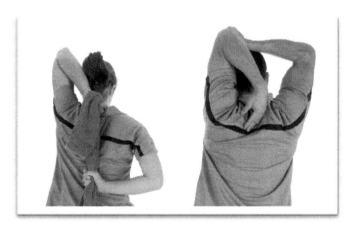

Stretch 2 – Assisted Triceps Stretch:
Stand with one hand behind your neck and your elbow pointing upwards. Then use your other hand (or a rope or towel) to pull your elbow down.

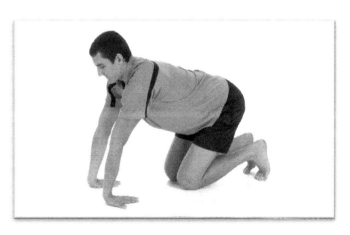

Stretch 3 – Kneeling Forearm Stretch:
While crouching on your knees with your forearms facing forward and hands pointing backwards, slowly move rearward.

Stretching Routine for
Elbow Sprain #2

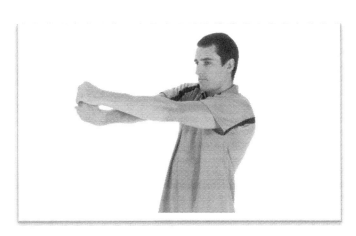

Stretch 1 – Rotating Wrist Stretch: Place one arm straight out in front and parallel to the ground. Rotate your wrist down and outwards and then use your other hand to further rotate your hand upwards.

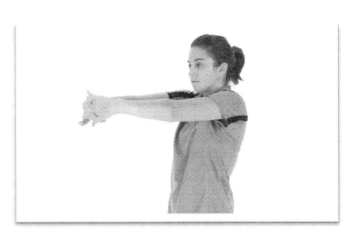

Stretch 2 – Palms-out Forearm Stretch: Interlock your fingers in front of your chest, then straighten your arms and turn the palms of your hands so that they face outwards.

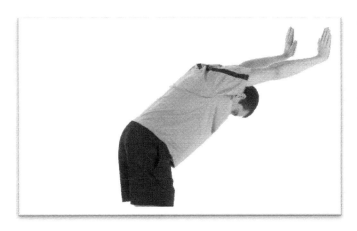

Stretch 3 – Bent-over Chest Stretch: Face a wall and place both hands on the wall just above your head. Slowly lower your shoulders as if moving your chin towards the ground.

Stretching Routine for
Triceps Tendon Rupture #1

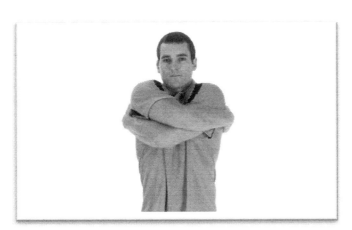

Stretch 1 – Wrap-around Shoulder
Stretch: Stand upright and wrap your arms around your shoulders as if hugging yourself. Pull your shoulders back.

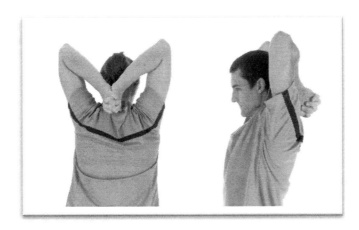

Stretch 2 – Reaching-down Triceps
Stretch: Reach behind your head with both hands and your elbows pointing upwards. Then reach down your back with your hands.

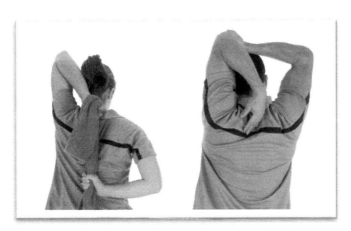

Stretch 3 – Assisted Triceps Stretch:
Stand with one hand behind your neck and your elbow pointing upwards. Then use your other hand (or a rope or towel) to pull your elbow down.

Stretching Routine for
Triceps Tendon Rupture #2

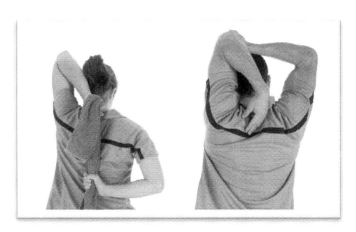

Stretch 1 – Assisted Triceps Stretch:
Stand with one hand behind your neck and your elbow pointing upwards. Then use your other hand (or a rope or towel) to pull your elbow down.

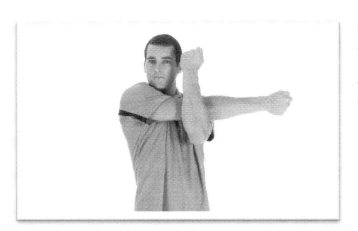

Stretch 2 – Parallel Arm Shoulder
Stretch: Stand upright and place one arm across your body. Keep your arm parallel to the ground and pull your elbow towards your body.

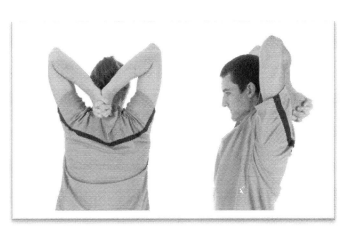

Stretch 3 – Reaching-down Triceps
Stretch: Reach behind your head with both hands and your elbows pointing upwards. Then reach down your back with your hands.

Stretching Routine for
Tennis, Golfers & Throwers Elbow #1

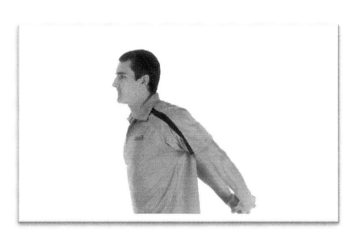

Stretch 1 – Reverse Shoulder Stretch:
Stand upright and clasp your hands together behind your back. Keep your arms straight and slowly lift your hands upward.

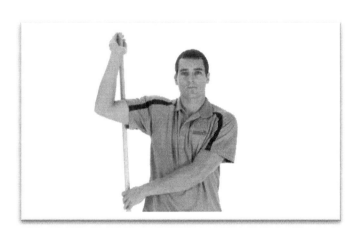

Stretch 2 – Arm-up Rotator Stretch:
Stand with your arm out and your forearm pointing upwards at 90 degrees. Place a broom stick in your hand and behind your elbow. With your other hand pull the bottom of the broom stick forward.

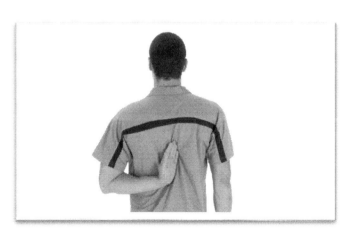

Stretch 3 – Reaching-up Shoulder Stretch:
Place one hand behind your back and then reach up between your shoulder blades.

Stretching Routine for
Tennis, Golfers & Throwers Elbow #2

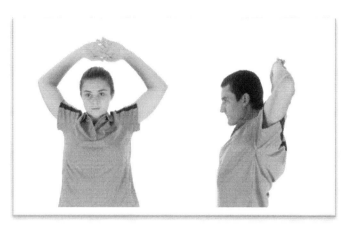

Stretch 1 – Above Head Chest Stretch:
Stand upright and interlock your fingers. Bend your arms and place them above your head while forcing your elbows and hands backwards.

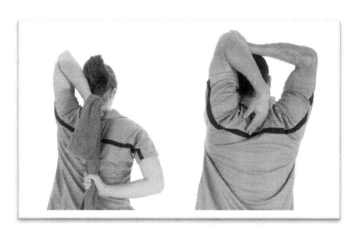

Stretch 2 – Assisted Triceps Stretch:
Stand with one hand behind your neck and your elbow pointing upwards. Then use your other hand (or a rope or towel) to pull your elbow down.

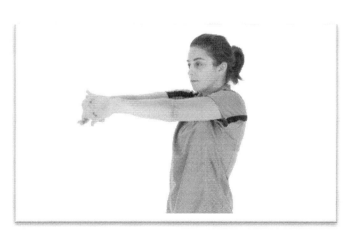

Stretch 3 – Palms-out Forearm Stretch:
Interlock your fingers in front of your chest, then straighten your arms and turn the palms of your hands so that they face outwards.

Stretching Routine for
Biceps Bruise, Strain & Tendinitis #1

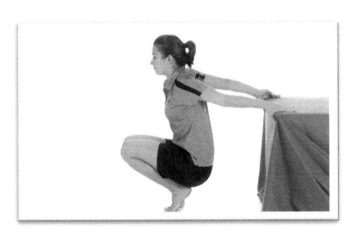

Stretch 1 – Assisted Reverse Shoulder
Stretch: Stand upright with your back towards a table or bench and place your hands on the edge of the table or bench. Keep your arms straight and slowly lower your entire body.

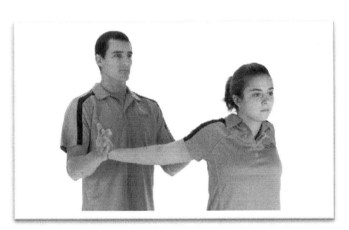

Stretch 2 – Partner Assisted Chest
Stretch: Extend both arms parallel to the ground and have a partner hold on to your hands, then slowly pull your arms backwards.

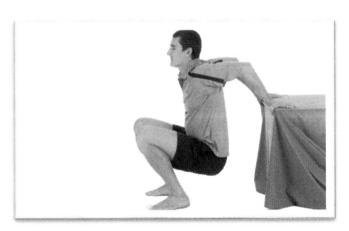

Stretch 3 – Assisted Reverse Chest
Stretch: Stand upright with your back towards a table or bench and place your hands on the edge of the table or bench. Bend your arms and slowly lower your entire body.

Stretching Routine for
Biceps Bruise, Strain & Tendinitis #2

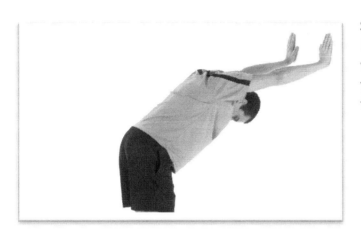

Stretch 1 – Bent-over Chest Stretch:
Face a wall and place both hands on the wall just above your head. Slowly lower your shoulders as if moving your chin towards the ground.

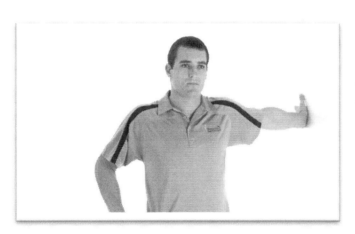

Stretch 2 – Parallel Arm Chest Stretch:
Stand with your arm extended to the rear and parallel to the ground. Hold on to an immovable object and then turn your shoulders and body away from your outstretched arm.

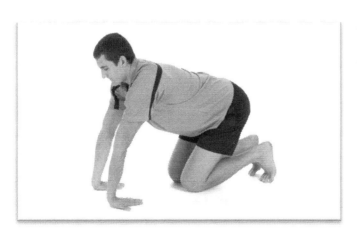

Stretch 3 – Kneeling Forearm Stretch:
While crouching on your knees with your forearms facing forward and hands pointing backwards, slowly move rearward.

Stretching Routine for Chest Strain #1

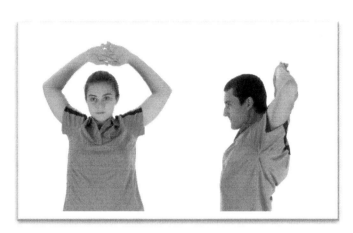

Stretch 1 – Above Head Chest Stretch:
Stand upright and interlock your fingers. Bend your arms and place them above your head while forcing your elbows and hands backwards.

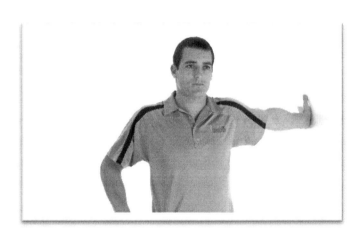

Stretch 2 – Parallel Arm Chest Stretch:
Stand with your arm extended to the rear and parallel to the ground. Hold on to an immovable object and then turn your shoulders and body away from your outstretched arm.

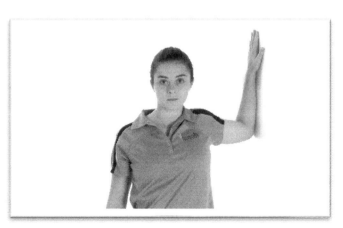

Stretch 3 – Bent Arm Chest Stretch:
Stand with your arm extended and your forearm pointing up at 90 degrees. Rest your forearm against an immovable object and then turn your shoulders and body away from your extended arm.

Stretching Routine for
Chest Strain #2

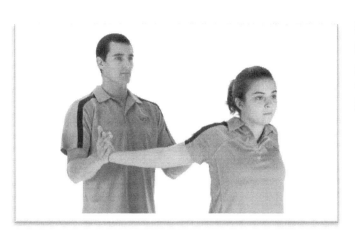

Stretch 1 – Partner Assisted Chest Stretch: Extend both arms parallel to the ground and have a partner hold on to your hands, then slowly pull your arms backwards.

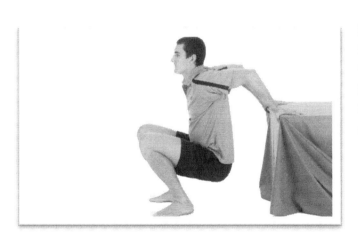

Stretch 2 – Assisted Reverse Chest Stretch: Stand upright with your back towards a table or bench and place your hands on the edge of the table or bench. Bend your arms and slowly lower your entire body.

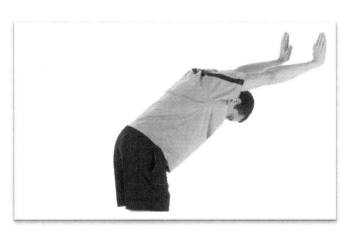

Stretch 3 – Bent-over Chest Stretch: Face a wall and place both hands on the wall just above your head. Slowly lower your shoulders as if moving your chin towards the ground.

Stretching Routine for
Pectoral Muscle Insertion Inflammation #1

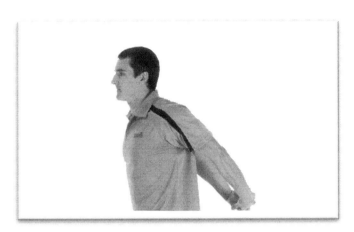

Stretch 1 – Reverse Shoulder Stretch:
Stand upright and clasp your hands together behind your back. Keep your arms straight and slowly lift your hands upward.

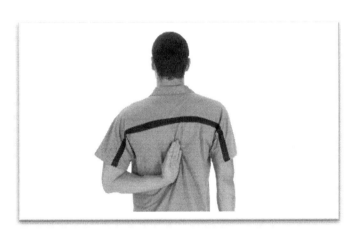

Stretch 2 – Reaching-up Shoulder Stretch: Place one hand behind your back and then reach up between your shoulder blades.

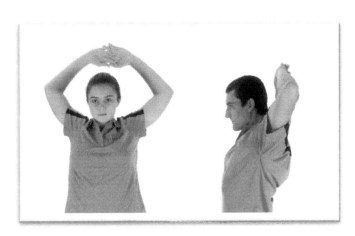

Stretch 3 –Above Head Chest Stretch:
Stand upright and interlock your fingers. Bend your arms and place them above your head while forcing your elbows and hands backwards.

Stretching Routine for
Pectoral Muscle Insertion Inflammation #2

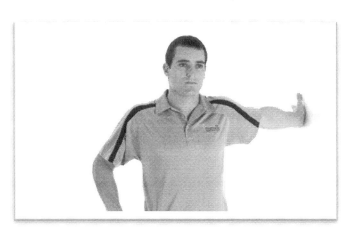

Stretch 1 – Parallel Arm Chest Stretch: Stand with your arm extended to the rear and parallel to the ground. Hold on to an immovable object and then turn your shoulders and body away from your outstretched arm.

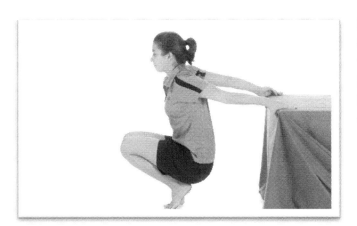

Stretch 2 – Assisted Reverse Shoulder Stretch: Stand upright with your back towards a table or bench and place your hands on the edge of the table or bench. Keep your arms straight and slowly lower your entire body.

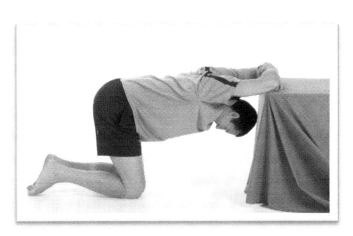

Stretch 3 – Kneeling Chest Stretch: Kneel on the floor in front of a chair or table and interlock your forearms above your head. Place your arms on the object and lower your upper body toward the ground.

Stretching Routine for
Shoulder Impingement Syndrome #1

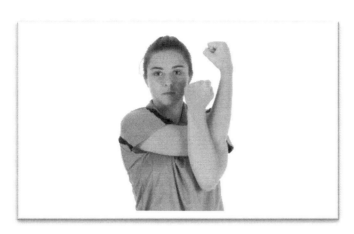

Stretch 1 – Bent Arm Shoulder Stretch:
Stand upright and place one arm across
your body. Bend your arm at 90 degrees
and pull your elbow towards your body.

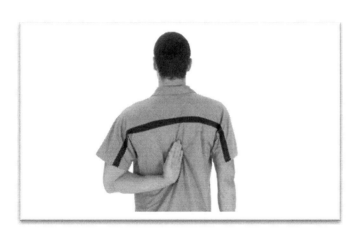

**Stretch 2 – Reaching-up Shoulder
Stretch:** Place one hand behind your
back and then reach up between your
shoulder blades.

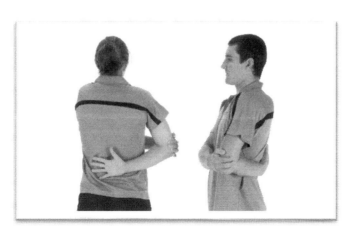

Stretch 3 –Elbow-out Rotator Stretch:
Stand with your hand behind the middle
of your back and your elbow pointing
out. Reach over with your other hand
and gently pull your elbow forward.

Stretching Routine for Shoulder Impingement Syndrome #2

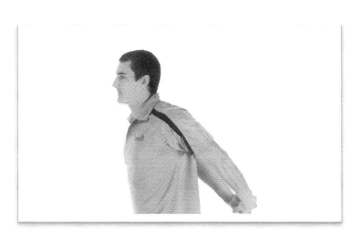

Stretch 1 – Reverse Shoulder Stretch:
Stand upright and clasp your hands together behind your back. Keep your arms straight and slowly lift your hands upward.

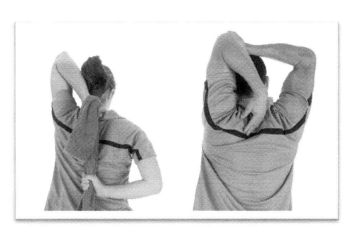

Stretch 2 – Assisted Triceps Stretch:
Stand with one hand behind your neck and your elbow pointing upwards. Then use your other hand (or a rope or towel) to pull your elbow down.

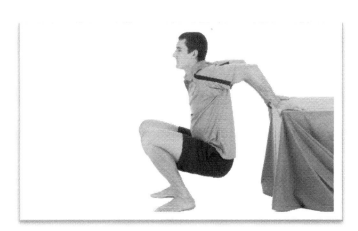

Stretch 3 – Assisted Reverse Chest Stretch: Stand upright with your back towards a table or bench and place your hands on the edge of the table or bench. Bend your arms and slowly lower your entire body.

Stretching Routine for
Rotator Cuff Tendinitis #1

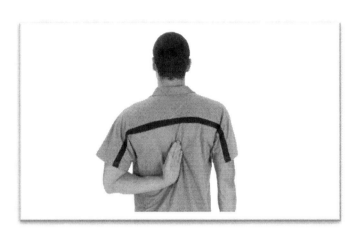

Stretch 1 – Reaching-up Shoulder Stretch: Place one hand behind your back and then reach up between your shoulder blades.

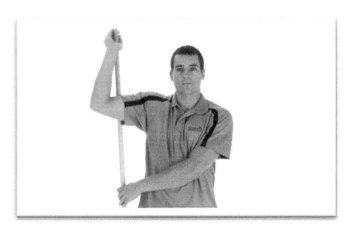

Stretch 2 – Arm-up Rotator Stretch: Stand with your arm out and your forearm pointing upwards at 90 degrees. Place a broom stick in your hand and behind your elbow. With your other hand pull the bottom of the broom stick forward.

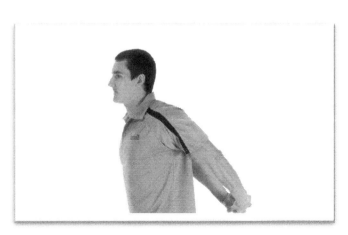

Stretch 3 – Reverse Shoulder Stretch: Stand upright and clasp your hands together behind your back. Keep your arms straight and slowly lift your hands upward.

Stretching Routine for Rotator Cuff Tendinitis #2

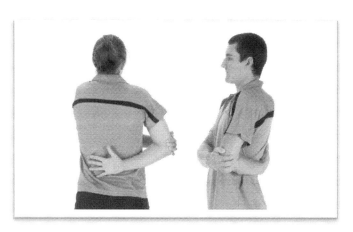

Stretch 1 – Elbow-out Rotator Stretch:
Stand with your hand behind the middle of your back and your elbow pointing out. Reach over with your other hand and gently pull your elbow forward.

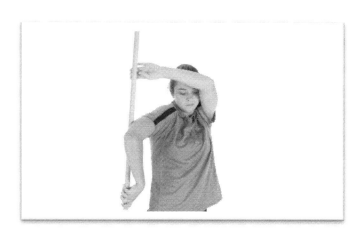

Stretch 2 – Arm-down Rotator Stretch:
Stand with your arm out and your forearm pointing downwards at 90 degrees. Place a broom stick in your hand and behind your elbow. With your other hand pull the top of the broom stick forward.

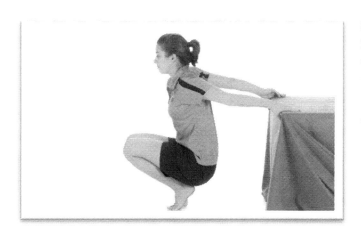

Stretch 3 – Assisted Reverse Shoulder Stretch:
Stand upright with your back towards a table or bench and place your hands on the edge of the table or bench. Keep your arms straight and slowly lower your entire body.

Stretching Routine for
Frozen Shoulder (Adhesive Capsulitis) #1

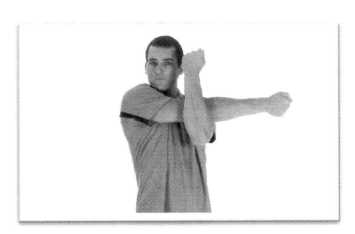

Stretch 1 – Parallel Arm Shoulder Stretch: Stand upright and place one arm across your body. Keep your arm parallel to the ground and pull your elbow towards your body.

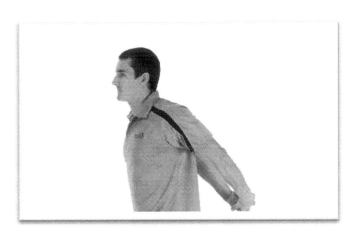

Stretch 2 – Reverse Shoulder Stretch: Stand upright and clasp your hands together behind your back. Keep your arms straight and slowly lift your hands upward.

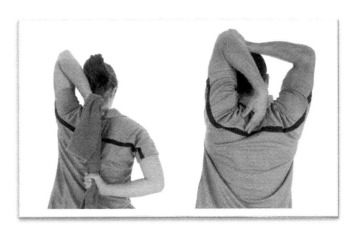

Stretch 3 – Assisted Triceps Stretch: Stand with one hand behind your neck and your elbow pointing upwards. Then use your other hand (or a rope or towel) to pull your elbow down.

Stretching Routine for
Frozen Shoulder (Adhesive Capsulitis) #2

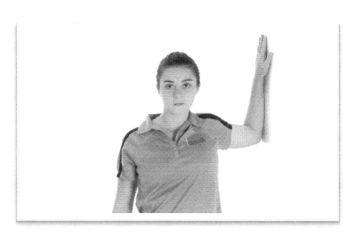

Stretch 1 – Bent Arm Chest Stretch:
Stand with your arm extended and your forearm pointing up at 90 degrees. Rest your forearm against an immovable object and then turn your shoulders and body away from your extended arm.

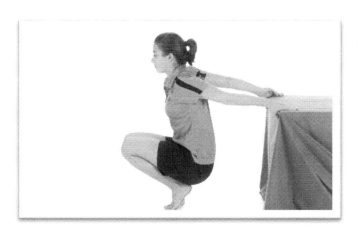

Stretch 2 – Assisted Reverse Shoulder Stretch:
Stand upright with your back towards a table or bench and place your hands on the edge of the table or bench. Keep your arms straight and slowly lower your entire body.

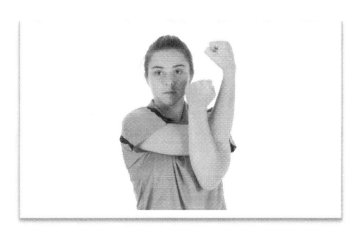

Stretch 3 – Bent Arm Shoulder Stretch:
Stand upright and place one arm across your body. Bend your arm at 90 degrees and pull your elbow towards your body.

Stretching Routine for
Back Muscle Bruise & Strain #1

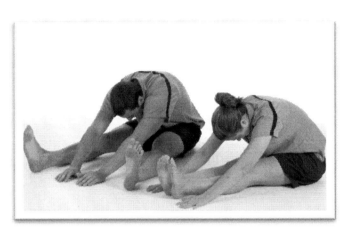

Stretch 1 – Sitting Bent-over Back Stretch: Sit on the ground with your legs straight out in front or at 45 degrees apart. Keep your toes pointing upwards and rest your arms by your side or on your lap. Relax your back and neck and let your head and chest fall forward.

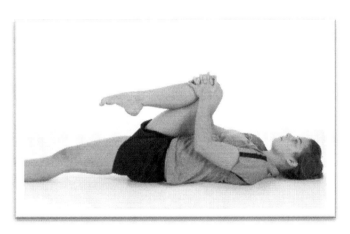

Stretch 2 –Lying Knee-to-chest Stretch: Lie on your back and keep one leg flat on the ground. Use your hands to bring your other knee into your chest.

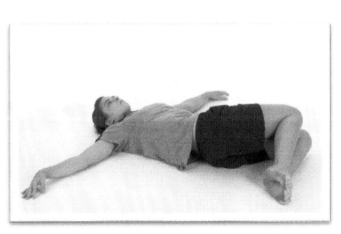

Stretch 3 – Lying Knee Roll-over Stretch: While lying on your back, bend your knees and let them fall to one side. Keep your arms out to the side and let your back and hips rotate with your knees.

Stretching Routine for Back Muscle Bruise & Strain #2

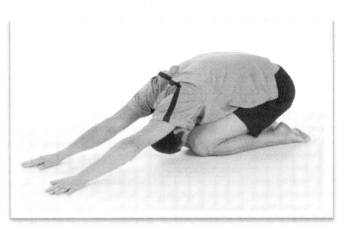

Stretch 1 –Kneeling Reach Forward Stretch: Kneel on the ground and reach forward with your hands. Let your head fall forward and push your buttocks back towards your feet.

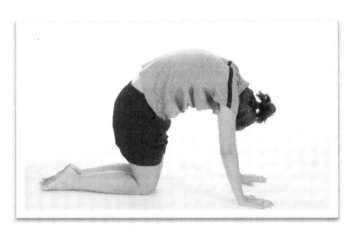

Stretch 2 – Kneeling Back-arch Stretch: Kneel on your hands and knees. Let your head fall forward and arch your back upwards.

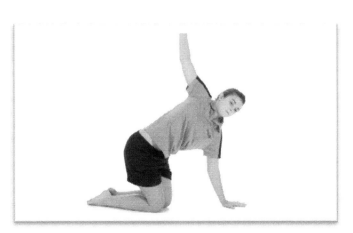

Stretch 3 – Kneeling Back Rotation Stretch: Kneel on the ground and raise one arm upwards while rotating your shoulders and middle back.

Stretching Routine for
Back Ligament Sprain #1

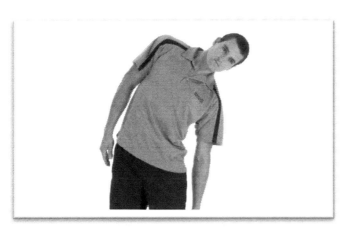

Stretch 1 –Standing Lateral Side Stretch: Stand with your feet about shoulder width apart and look forward. Keep your body upright and slowly bend to the left or right. Reach down your leg with your hand and do not bend forward.

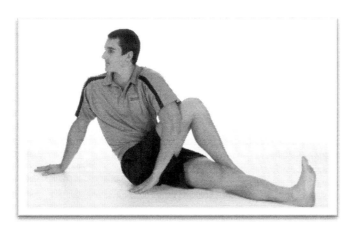

Stretch 2 – Sitting Knee-up Rotation Stretch: Sit with one leg straight and the other leg crossed over your knee. Turn your shoulders and put your arm onto your raised knee to help rotate your shoulders and back.

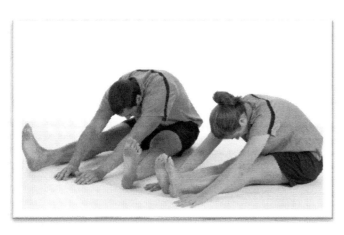

Stretch 3 – Sitting Bent-over Back Stretch: Sit on the ground with your legs straight out in front or at 45 degrees apart. Keep your toes pointing upwards and rest your arms by your side or on your lap. Relax your back and neck and let your head and chest fall forward.

Stretching Routine for Back Ligament Sprain #2

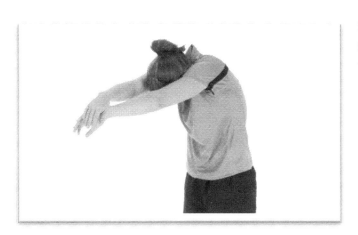

Stretch 1 – Reach Forward Upper Back Stretch: Stand with your arms out in front and your hands crossed over, then push your hands forward as far as possible and let your head fall forward.

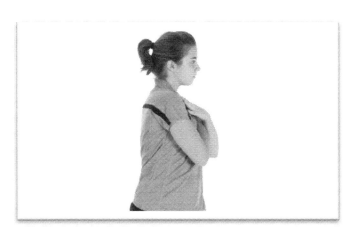

Stretch 2 – Standing Back Rotation Stretch: Stand with your feet shoulder width apart. Place your hands across your chest while keeping your back and shoulders upright. Slowly rotate your shoulders to one side.

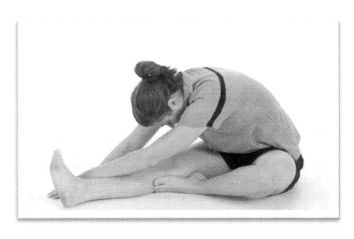

Stretch 3 –Sitting Side Reach Stretch: Sit with one leg straight out to the side and your toes pointing upwards. Then bring your other foot up to your knee and let your head fall forward. Reach towards the outside of your toes with both hands.

Stretching Routine for Abdominal Muscle Strain #1

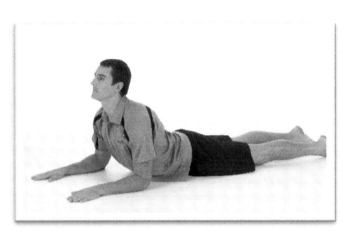

Stretch 1 – On Elbows Stomach Stretch: Lie face down and bring your hands close to your shoulders. Keep your hips on the ground, look forward and rise up onto your elbows.

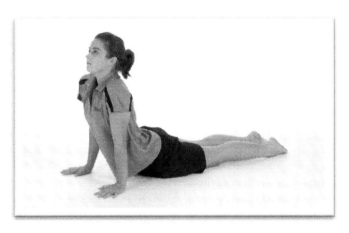

Stretch 2 – Rising Stomach Stretch: Lie face down and bring your hands close to your shoulders. Keep your hips on the ground, look forward and rise up by straightening your arms.

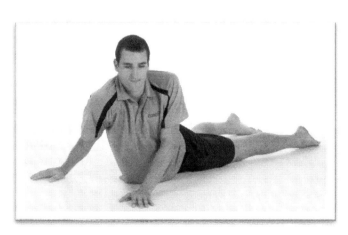

Stretch 3 – Rotating Stomach Stretch: Lie face down and bring your hands close to your shoulders. Keep your hips on the ground, look forward and rise up by straightening your arms. Then slowly bend one arm and rotate that shoulder towards the ground.

Stretching Routine for
Abdominal Muscle Strain #2

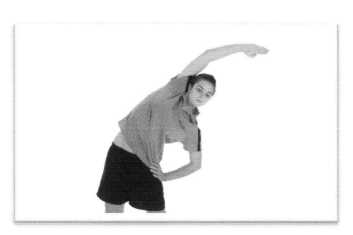

Stretch 1 – Reaching Lateral Side Stretch: Stand with your feet shoulder width apart, then slowly bend to the side and reach over the top of your head with your hand. Do not bend forward.

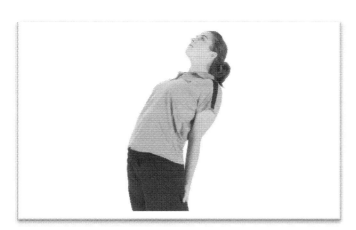

Stretch 2 – Standing Lean-back Stomach Stretch: Stand upright with your feet shoulder width apart and place your hands on your buttocks for support. Look upwards and slowly lean backwards at the waist.

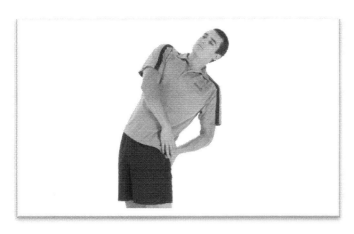

Stretch 3 – Standing Lean-back Side Stomach Stretch: Stand upright with your feet shoulder width apart and place one hand of your buttocks. Look up and slowly lean backwards at the waist, then reach over with your opposite hand and rotate at the waist.

Stretching Routine for
Hip Flexor Strain & Iliopsoas Tendinitis #1

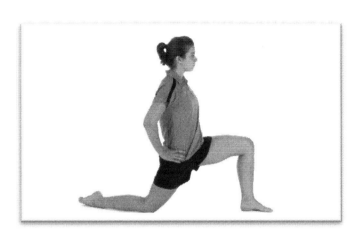

Stretch 1 – Kneeling Quad Stretch: Kneel on one foot and the other knee. If needed, hold on to something to keep your balance and then push your hips forward.

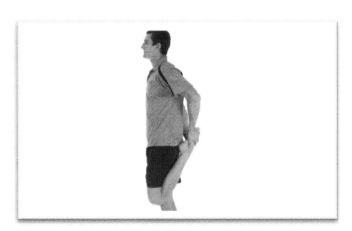

Stretch 2 – Standing Quad Stretch: Stand upright while balancing on one leg. Pull your other foot up behind your buttocks and keep your knees together while pushing your hips forward. Hold on to something for balance if needed.

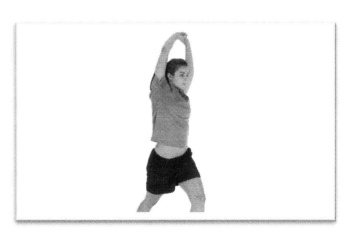

Stretch 3 – Standing Reach-up Quad Stretch: Stand upright and take one small step forward. Reach up with both hands, push your hips forward, lean back and then lean away from your back leg.

Stretching Routine for
Hip Flexor Strain & Iliopsoas Tendinitis #2

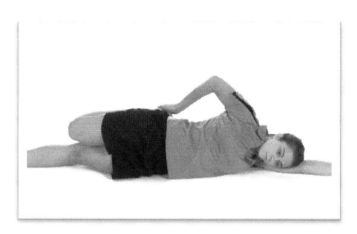

Stretch 1 – Lying Side Quad Stretch: Lie on your side and pull your top leg behind your buttocks. Keep your knees together and push your hips forward.

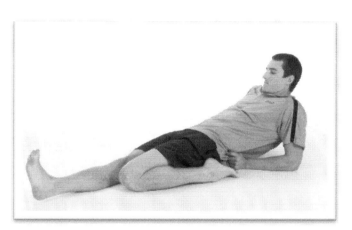

Stretch 2 – Single Lean-back Quad Stretch: Sit on the ground, bend one knee and place that foot next to your buttocks. Then slowly lean backwards.

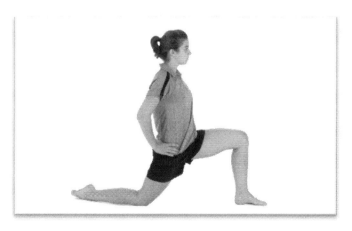

Stretch 3 – Kneeling Quad Stretch: Kneel on one foot and the other knee. If needed, hold on to something to keep your balance and then push your hips forward.

Stretching Routine for
Groin Strain & Tendinitis #1

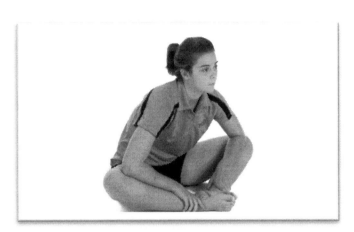

Stretch 1 – Sitting Feet-together Adductor Stretch: Sit with the soles of your feet together and bring your feet towards your groin. Hold onto your ankles and push your knees toward the ground with your elbows. Keep your back straight.

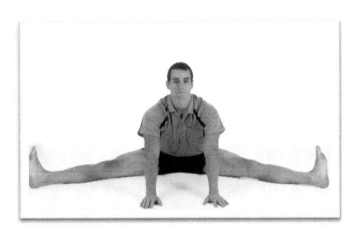

Stretch 2 –Sitting Wide-leg Adductor Stretch: Sit on the ground with your legs straight out and as wide apart as possible and then reach forward while keeping your back straight.

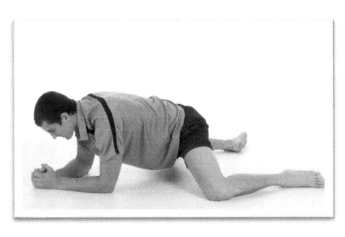

Stretch 3 –Kneeling Face-down Adductor Stretch: Kneel face down with your knees and toes facing out. Lean forward and let your knees move outwards.

Stretching Routine for
Groin Strain & Tendinitis #2

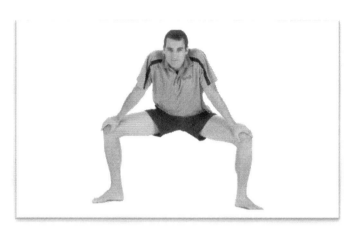

Stretch 1 – Standing Wide Knees Adductor Stretch: Stand with your feet wide apart and your toes pointing diagonally outwards, then bend your knees, lean forward and use your hands to push your knees outwards.

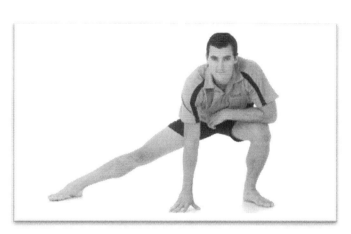

Stretch 2 – Squatting Leg-out Adductor Stretch: Stand with your feet wide apart. Keep one leg straight and your toes pointing forward while bending the other leg and turning your toes out to the side. Lower your groin towards the ground and rest your hands on your bent knee or the ground.

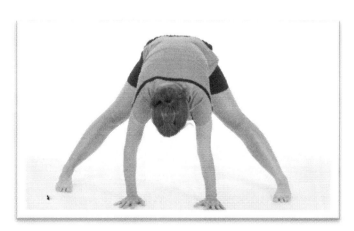

Stretch 3 – Standing Wide-leg Adductor Stretch: Start by standing with your feet wide apart and your toes pointing forward. Then lean forward and reach towards the ground.

Stretching Routine for Osteitis Pubis #1

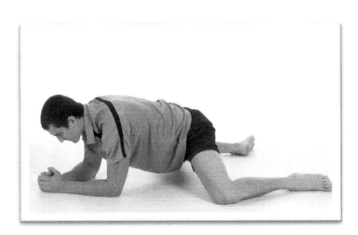

Stretch 1 – Kneeling Face-down Adductor Stretch: Kneel face down with your knees and toes facing out. Lean forward and let your knees move outwards.

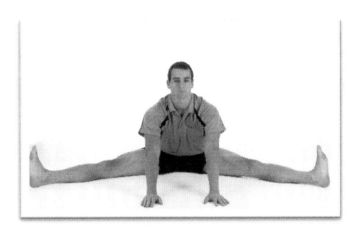

Stretch 2 – Sitting Wide-leg Adductor Stretch: Sit on the ground with your legs straight out and as wide apart as possible and then reach forward while keeping your back straight.

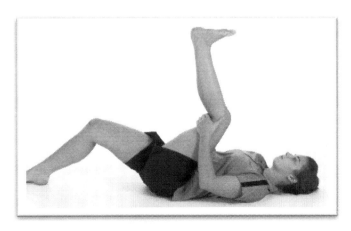

Stretch 3 – Lying Bent Knee Hamstring Stretch: Lie on your back and bend one leg slightly. Pull the other knee towards your chest and then slowly straighten your raised leg.

Stretching Routine for
Osteitis Pubis #2

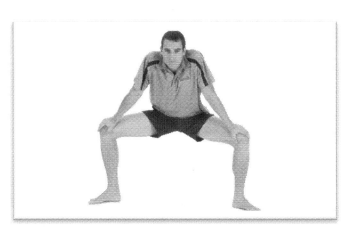

Stretch 1 – Standing Wide Knees Adductor Stretch: Stand with your feet wide apart and your toes pointing diagonally outwards, then bend your knees, lean forward and use your hands to push your knees outwards.

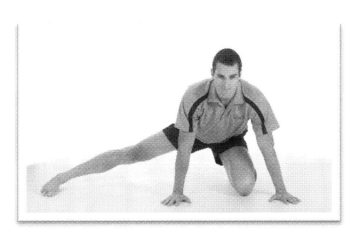

Stretch 2 – Kneeling Leg-out Adductor Stretch: Kneel on one knee and place your other leg out to the side with your toes pointing forward. Rest your hands on the ground and slowly move your foot further out to the side.

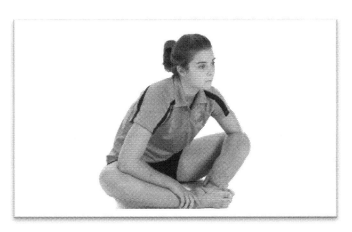

Stretch 3 – Sitting Feet-together Adductor Stretch: Sit with the soles of your feet together and bring your feet towards your groin. Hold onto your ankles and push your knees toward the ground with your elbows. Keep your back straight.

Stretching Routine for
Piriformis Syndrome #1

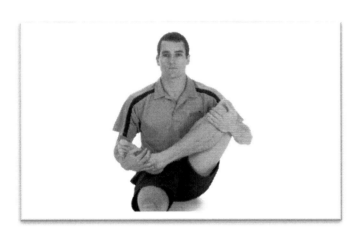

Stretch 1 – Sitting Foot-to-chest Buttocks Stretch: Sit with one leg straight, hold onto your other ankle and then pull it directly towards your chest.

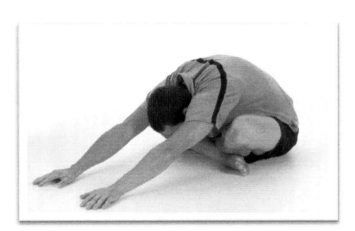

Stretch 2 – Sitting Cross-legged Reach Forward Stretch: Sit with your legs crossed and your knees out, and then gently reach forward.

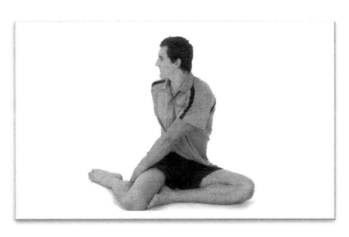

Stretch 3 – Sitting Rotational Hip Stretch: Sit with one leg crossed and your other leg behind your buttocks then lean your whole body towards the leg that is behind your buttocks.

Stretching Routine for Piriformis Syndrome #2

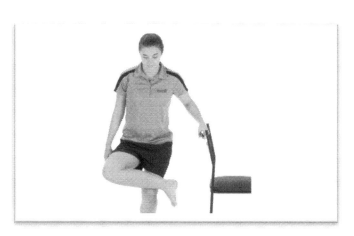

Stretch 1 – Standing Leg Resting Hip Stretch: Stand beside a chair or table for balance, bend one leg and place your other ankle on to your bent knee. Slowly lower yourself towards the ground.

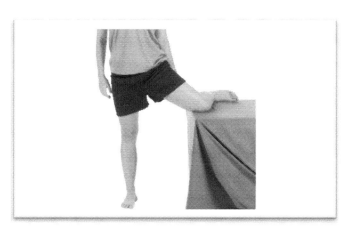

Stretch 2 – Standing Rotational Hip Stretch: Stand beside a table and raise your lower leg out to the side and up onto the table. Then slowly lower your body.

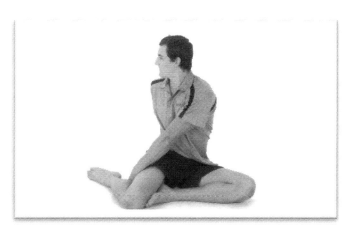

Stretch 3 – Sitting Rotational Hip Stretch: Sit with one leg crossed and your other leg behind your buttocks then lean your whole body towards the leg that is behind your buttocks.

Stretching Routine for
Quadriceps Bruise, Strain & Tendinitis #1

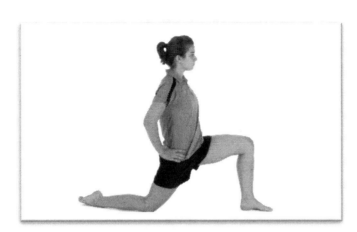

Stretch 1 – Kneeling Quad Stretch: Kneel on one foot and the other knee. If needed, hold on to something to keep your balance and then push your hips forward.

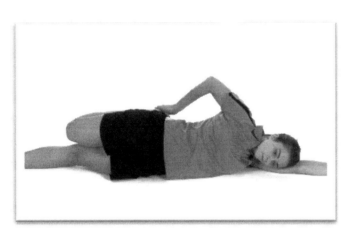

Stretch 2 – Lying Side Quad Stretch: Lie on your side and pull your top leg behind your buttocks. Keep your knees together and push your hips forward.

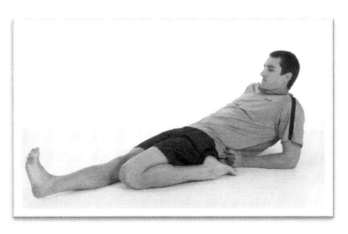

Stretch 3 – Single Lean-back Quad Stretch: Sit on the ground, bend one knee and place that foot next to your buttocks. Then slowly lean backwards.

Stretching Routine for
Quadriceps Bruise, Strain & Tendinitis #2

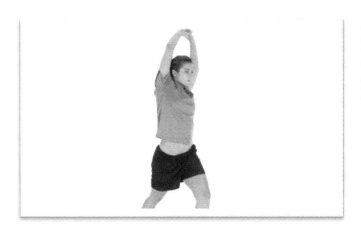

Stretch 1 – Standing Reach-up Quad Stretch: Stand upright and take one small step forward. Reach up with both hands, push your hips forward, lean back and then lean away from your back leg.

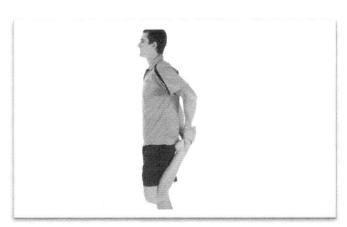

Stretch 2 – Standing Quad Stretch: Stand upright while balancing on one leg. Pull your other foot up behind your buttocks and keep your knees together while pushing your hips forward. Hold on to something for balance if needed.

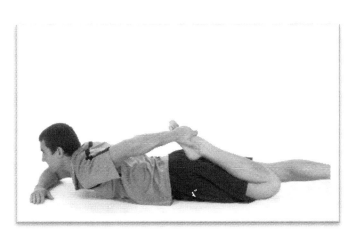

Stretch 3 – Lying Quad Stretch: Lie face down, reach back with one hand and pull one foot up behind your buttocks.

Stretching Routine for
Hamstring Strain #1

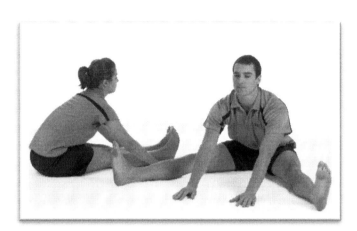

Stretch 1 – Sitting Reach-forward Hamstring Stretch: Sit with both legs straight out in front, or at 45 degrees apart. Keep your toes pointing straight up, make sure your back is straight and then reach forward.

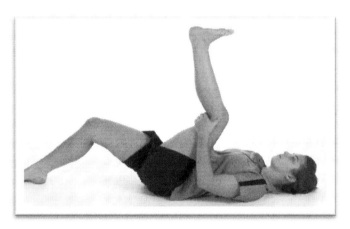

Stretch 2 – Lying Bent Knee Hamstring Stretch: Lie on your back and bend one leg slightly. Pull the other knee towards your chest and then slowly straighten your raised leg.

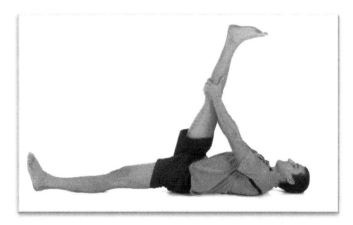

Stretch 3 – Lying Straight Knee Hamstring Stretch: Lie on your back and keep your legs straight. Raise one leg and pull it towards your chest.

Stretching Routine for Hamstring Strain #2

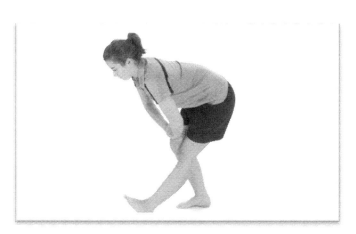

Stretch 1 –Standing Toe-up Hamstring Stretch: Stand with one knee bent and the other leg straight out in front. Point your toes upwards and lean forward. Keep your back straight and rest your hands on your bent knee.

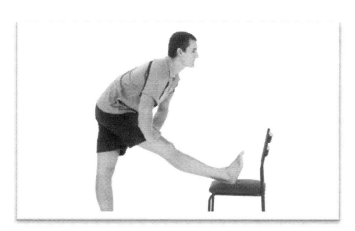

Stretch 2 – Standing Leg-up Hamstring Stretch: Stand upright and raise one leg on to an object. Keep that leg straight and point your toes upwards. Keep your back straight and lean your upper body forward.

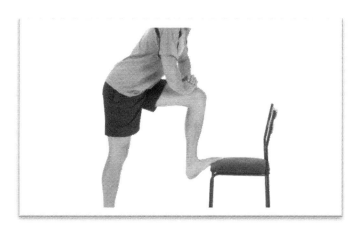

Stretch 3 – Standing Leg-up Bent Knee Hamstring Stretch: Stand with one foot raised onto a chair or an object. Bend your knee and let your heel drop off the edge of the object. Keep your back straight and move your chest towards your raised knee.

Stretching Routine for
Iliotibial Band Syndrome #1

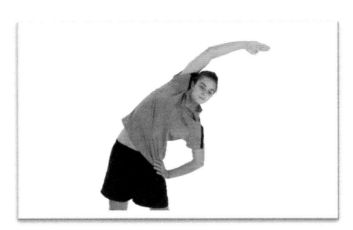

Stretch 1 – Reaching Lateral Side
Stretch: Stand with your feet shoulder width apart, then slowly bend to the side and reach over the top of your head with your hand. Do not bend forward.

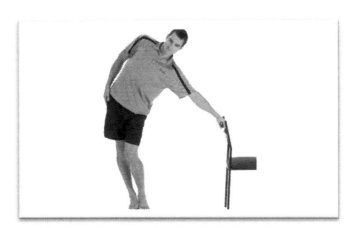

Stretch 2 – Standing Hip-out Abductor
Stretch: Stand upright beside a chair or table with both feet together. Lean your upper body towards the chair while pushing your hips away from the chair. Keep your outside leg straight and bend your inside leg slightly.

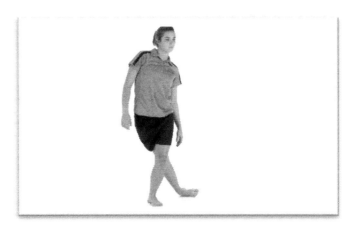

Stretch 3 – Standing Leg-cross Abductor
Stretch: Stand upright and cross one foot behind the other. Lean towards the foot that is behind the other.

Stretching Routine for
Iliotibial Band Syndrome #2

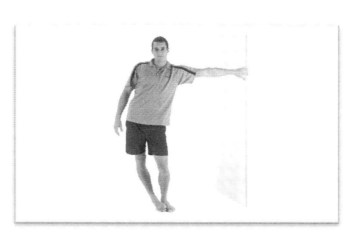

Stretch 1 – Leaning Abductor Stretch:
While standing next to a pole, or door jam, hold onto the pole with one hand. Keep your feet together, and lean your hips away from the pole. Keep your outside leg straight and bend your inside leg slightly.

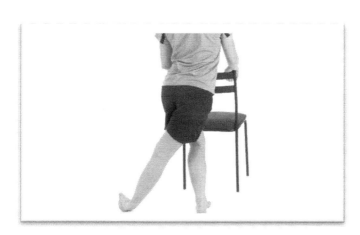

Stretch 2 – Standing Leg-under Abductor Stretch: While standing lean forward and hold onto a chair or bench to help with balance. Cross one foot behind the other and slide that foot to the side. Keep your leg straight and slowly bend your front leg to lower your body.

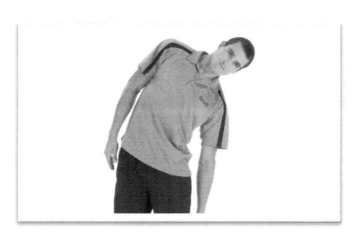

Stretch 3 – Standing Lateral Side Stretch:
Stand with your feet about shoulder width apart and look forward. Keep your body upright and slowly bend to the left or right. Reach down your leg with your hand and do not bend forward.

Stretching Routine for
Medial Collateral Ligament Sprain (MCL) #1

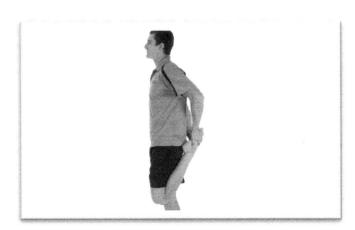

Stretch 1 – Standing Quad Stretch: Stand upright while balancing on one leg. Pull your other foot up behind your buttocks and keep your knees together while pushing your hips forward. Hold on to something for balance if needed.

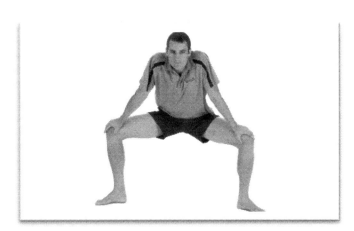

Stretch 2 – Standing Wide Knees Adductor Stretch: Stand with your feet wide apart and your toes pointing diagonally outwards, then bend your knees, lean forward and use your hands to push your knees outwards.

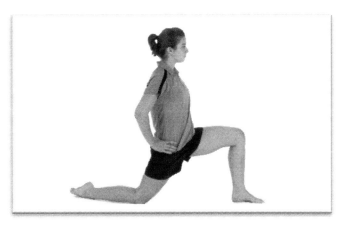

Stretch 3 – Kneeling Quad Stretch: Kneel on one foot and the other knee. If needed, hold on to something to keep your balance and then push your hips forward.

Stretching Routine for
Medial Collateral Ligament Sprain (MCL) #2

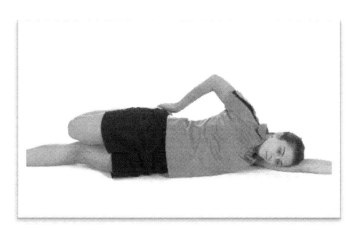

Stretch 1 – Lying Side Quad Stretch: Lie on your side and pull your top leg behind your buttocks. Keep your knees together and push your hips forward.

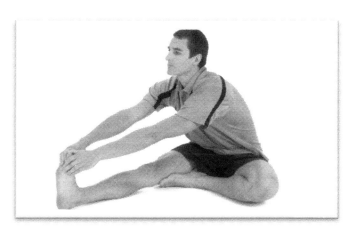

Stretch 2 – Sitting Single Leg Hamstring Stretch: Sit with one leg straight out in front and point your toes upwards. Bring your other foot towards your knee and reach towards your toes with both hands.

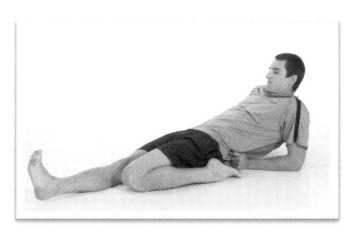

Stretch 3 – Single Lean-back Quad Stretch: Sit on the ground, bend one knee and place that foot next to your buttocks. Then slowly lean backwards.

Stretching Routine for
Anterior Cruciate Ligament Sprain (ACL) #1

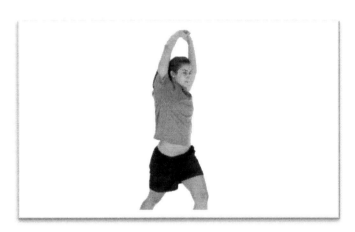

Stretch 1 – Standing Reach-up Quad Stretch: Stand upright and take one small step forward. Reach up with both hands, push your hips forward, lean back and then lean away from your back leg.

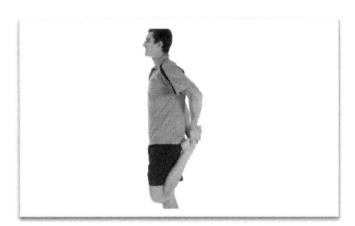

Stretch 2 – Standing Quad Stretch: Stand upright while balancing on one leg. Pull your other foot up behind your buttocks and keep your knees together while pushing your hips forward. Hold on to something for balance if needed.

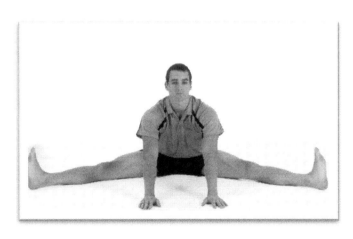

Stretch 3 – Sitting Wide-leg Adductor Stretch: Sit on the ground with your legs straight out and as wide apart as possible and then reach forward while keeping your back straight.

Stretching Routine for
Anterior Cruciate Ligament Sprain (ACL) #2

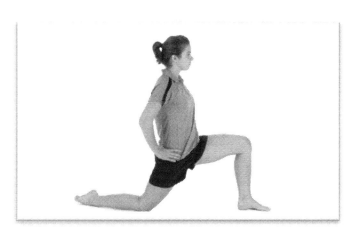

Stretch 1 – Kneeling Quad Stretch: Kneel on one foot and the other knee. If needed, hold on to something to keep your balance and then push your hips forward.

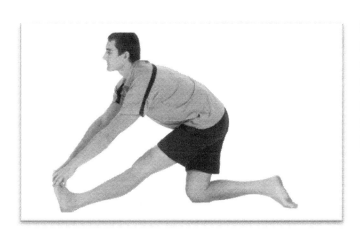

Stretch 2 – Kneeling Toe-up Hamstring Stretch: Kneel on one knee and place your other leg straight forward with your heel on the ground. Keep your back straight and point your toes upwards. Reach towards your toes with one or both hand.

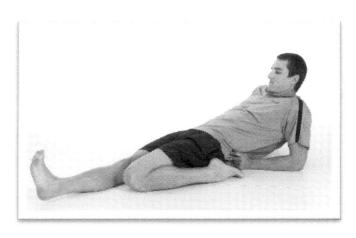

Stretch 3 – Single Lean-back Quad Stretch: Sit on the ground, bend one knee and place that foot next to your buttocks. Then slowly lean backwards.

Stretching Routine for
Osgood-Schlatter Syndrome #1

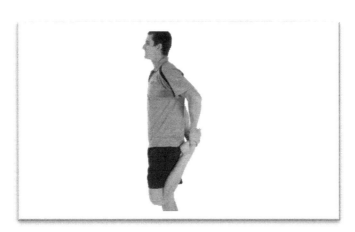

Stretch 1 – Standing Quad Stretch: Stand upright while balancing on one leg. Pull your other foot up behind your buttocks and keep your knees together while pushing your hips forward. Hold on to something for balance if needed.

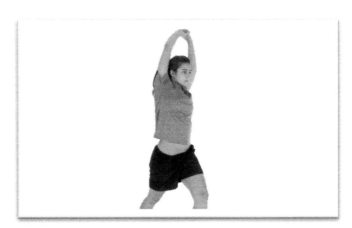

Stretch 2 – Standing Reach-up Quad Stretch: Stand upright and take one small step forward. Reach up with both hands, push your hips forward, lean back and then lean away from your back leg.

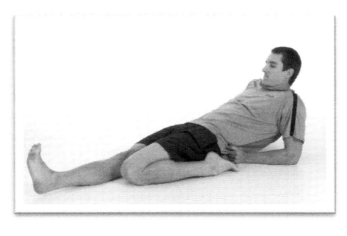

Stretch 3 – Single Lean-back Quad Stretch: Sit on the ground, bend one knee and place that foot next to your buttocks. Then slowly lean backwards.

Stretching Routine for Osgood-Schlatter Syndrome #2

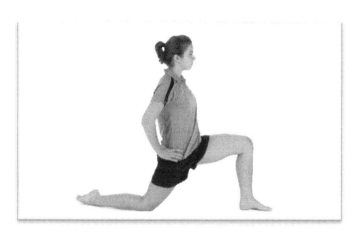

Stretch 1 – Kneeling Quad Stretch: Kneel on one foot and the other knee. If needed, hold on to something to keep your balance and then push your hips forward.

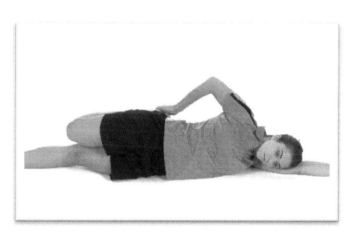

Stretch 2 – Lying Side Quad Stretch: Lie on your side and pull your top leg behind your buttocks. Keep your knees together and push your hips forward.

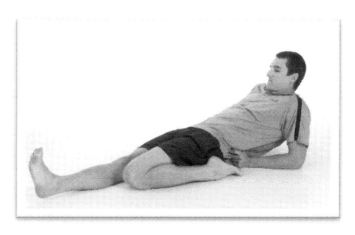

Stretch 3 – Single Lean-back Quad Stretch: Sit on the ground, bend one knee and place that foot next to your buttocks. Then slowly lean backwards.

Stretching Routine for Patellofemerol Pain Syndrome #1

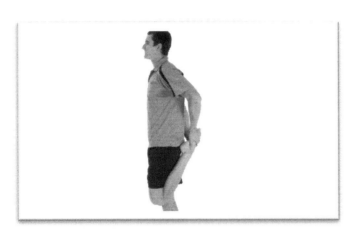

Stretch 1 – Standing Quad Stretch: Stand upright while balancing on one leg. Pull your other foot up behind your buttocks and keep your knees together while pushing your hips forward. Hold on to something for balance if needed.

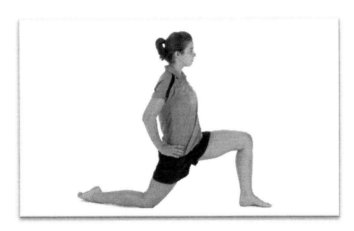

Stretch 2 – Kneeling Quad Stretch: Kneel on one foot and the other knee. If needed, hold on to something to keep your balance and then push your hips forward.

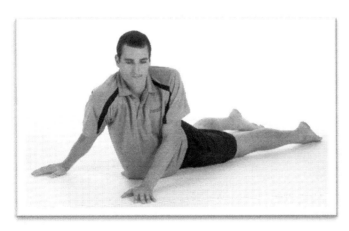

Stretch 3 – Rotating Hip Stretch: Lie face down and bring your hands close to your shoulders. Keep your hips on the ground, look forward and rise up by straightening your arms. Then slowly bend one arm and rotate that shoulder towards the ground.

Stretching Routine for Patellofemerol Pain Syndrome #2

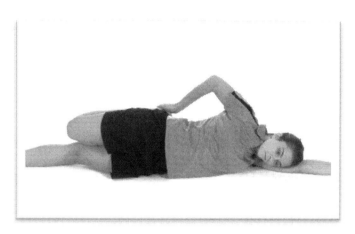

Stretch 1 – Lying Side Quad Stretch: Lie on your side and pull your top leg behind your buttocks. Keep your knees together and push your hips forward.

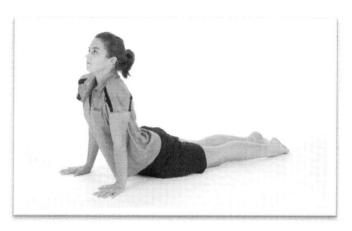

Stretch 2 – Rising Stomach Stretch: Lie face down and bring your hands close to your shoulders. Keep your hips on the ground, look forward and rise up by straightening your arms.

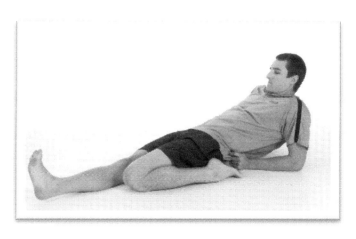

Stretch 3 – Single Lean-back Quad Stretch: Sit on the ground, bend one knee and place that foot next to your buttocks. Then slowly lean backwards.

Stretching Routine for
Patellar Tendinitis (Jumpers Knee) #1

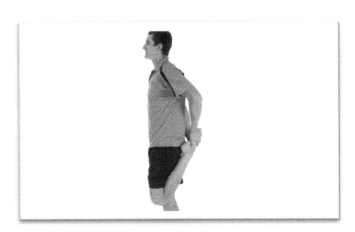

Stretch 1 – Standing Quad Stretch: Stand upright while balancing on one leg. Pull your other foot up behind your buttocks and keep your knees together while pushing your hips forward. Hold on to something for balance if needed.

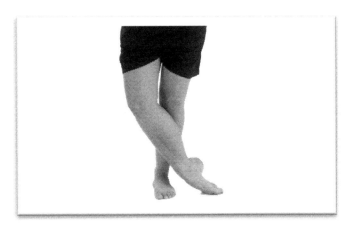

Stretch 2 – Front Cross-over Shin Stretch: Stand upright and place the top of your toes on the ground in front of your other foot. Slowly bend your other knee to force your ankle to the ground.

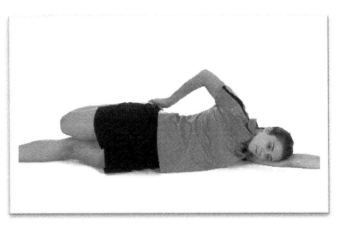

Stretch 3 – Lying Side Quad Stretch: Lie on your side and pull your top leg behind your buttocks. Keep your knees together and push your hips forward.

Stretching Routine for
Patellar Tendinitis (Jumpers Knee) #2

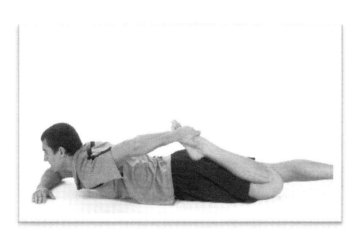

Stretch 1 – Lying Quad Stretch: Lie face down, reach back with one hand and pull one foot up behind your buttocks.

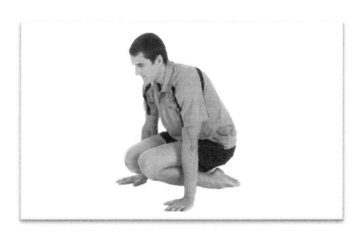

Stretch 2 – Double Kneeling Shin Stretch: Sit with your knees and feet flat on the ground. Sit back on your ankles and keep your knees together. Place your hands next to your knees and slowly lean backwards while raising your knees off the ground.

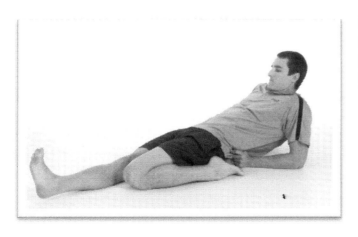

Stretch 3 – Single Lean-back Quad Stretch: Sit on the ground, bend one knee and place that foot next to your buttocks. Then slowly lean backwards.

Stretching Routine for
Calf Strain #1

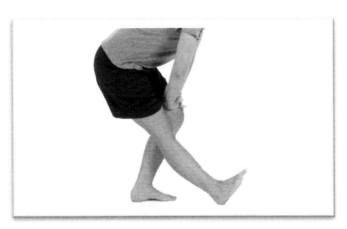

Stretch 1 – Standing Toe Raised Calf Stretch: Stand with one knee bent and the other leg straight out in front. Point your toes upwards and lean forward. Keep your back straight and rest your hands on your bent knee.

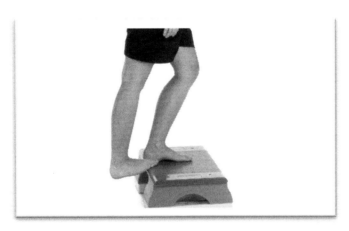

Stretch 2 – Single Heel-drop Calf Stretch: Stand on a raised object or step. Put the ball of one foot on the edge of the step and keep your leg straight. Let your heel drop towards the ground.

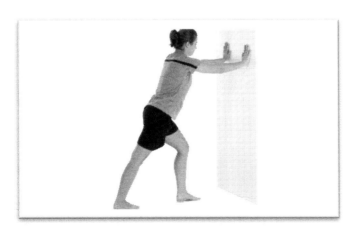

Stretch 3 – Leaning Heel-back Calf Stretch: Reach towards a wall and place one foot as far from the wall as is comfortable. Make sure that both toes are pointing forward and your heel is on the ground. Keep your back leg straight and lean towards the wall.

Stretching Routine for
Calf Strain #2

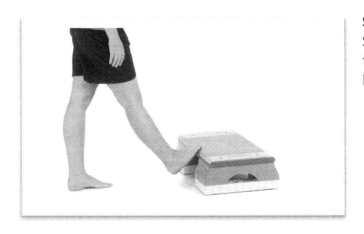

Stretch 1 – Standing Toe-up Calf Stretch:
Stand upright and place the ball of your foot on a step or raised object. Keep your leg straight and lean towards your toes.

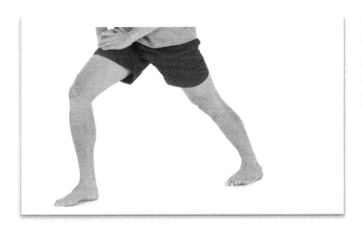

Stretch 2 – Standing Heel-back Calf Stretch: Stand upright and take one big step backwards. Keep your back leg straight, your toes pointing forward and push your heel to the ground.

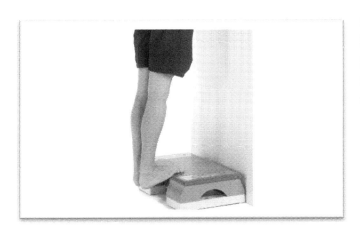

Stretch 3 – Double Heel-drop Calf Stretch: Stand on a raised object or step. Put the balls of both feet on the edge of the step and keep your legs straight. Let your heels drop towards the ground.

Stretching Routine for
Achilles Tendon Strain & Tendinitis #1

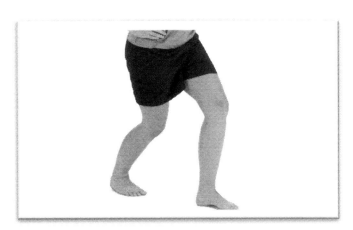

Stretch 1 – Standing Heel-back Achilles
Stretch: Stand upright and take one step backwards. Bend your back knee and push your heel towards the ground.

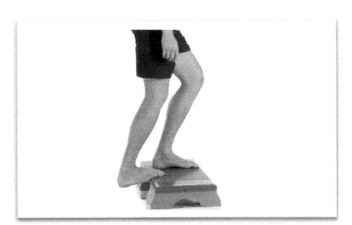

Stretch 2 – Single Heel-drop Achilles
Stretch: Stand on a raised object or step and place the ball of one of your feet on the edge of the step. Bend your knee slightly and let your heel drop towards the ground.

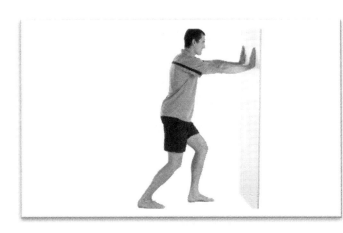

Stretch 3 – Leaning Heel-back Achilles
Stretch: Reach towards a wall and place one foot as far from the wall as is comfortable. Make sure that both toes are pointing forward and your heels are on the ground. Bend your back knee and lean towards the wall.

Stretching Routine for
Achilles Tendon Strain & Tendinitis #2

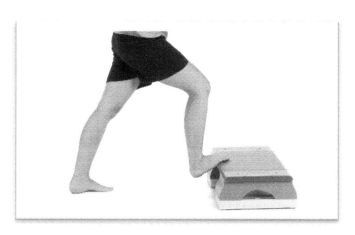

Stretch 1 – Standing Toe-up Achilles Stretch: Stand upright and place the ball of your foot onto a step or raised object. Bend your knee and lean forward.

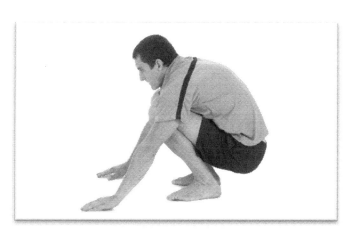

Stretch 2 – Squatting Achilles Stretch: Stand with your feet shoulder width apart. Then bend your legs and lower your body into a sitting position. Place your hands out in front for balance.

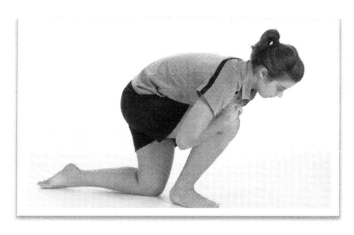

Stretch 3 – Kneeling Heel-down Achilles Stretch: Kneel on one foot and place your body weight over your knee. Keep your heel on the ground and lean forward.

Stretching Routine for
Shin Splints (MTSS) #1

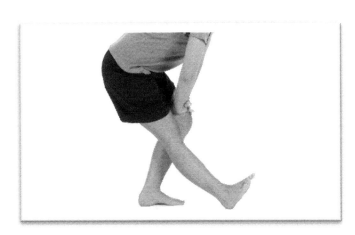

Stretch 1 – Standing Toe Raised Calf
Stretch: Stand with one knee bent and the other leg straight out in front. Point your toes upwards and lean forward. Keep your back straight and rest your hands on your bent knee.

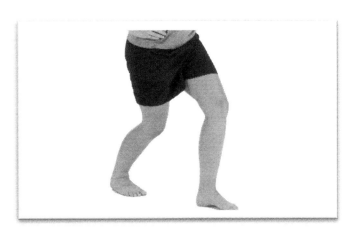

Stretch 2 – Standing Heel-back Achilles
Stretch: Stand upright and take one step backwards. Bend your back knee and push your heel towards the ground.

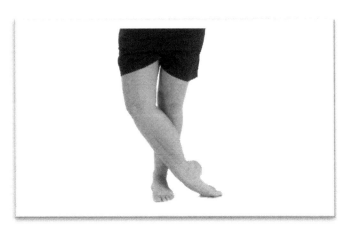

Stretch 3 –Front Cross-over Shin Stretch:
Stand upright and place the top of your toes on the ground in front of your other foot. Slowly bend your other knee to force your ankle to the ground.

Stretching Routine for Shin Splints (MTSS) #2

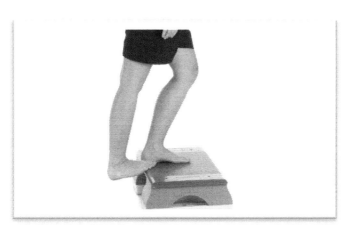

Stretch 1 – Single Heel-drop Calf Stretch: Stand on a raised object or step. Put the ball of one foot on the edge of the step and keep your leg straight. Let your heel drop towards the ground.

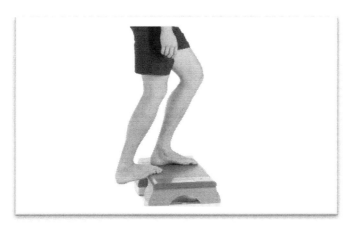

Stretch 2 – Single Heel-drop Achilles Stretch: Stand on a raised object or step and place the ball of one of your feet on the edge of the step. Bend your knee slightly and let your heel drop towards the ground.

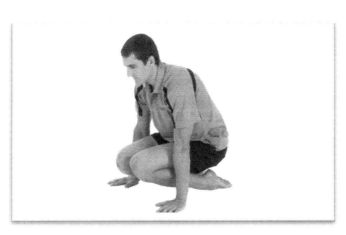

Stretch 3 – Double Kneeling Shin Stretch: Sit with your knees and feet flat on the ground. Sit back on your ankles and keep your knees together. Place your hands next to your knees and slowly lean backwards while raising your knees off the ground.

Stretching Routine for
Anterior Compartment Syndrome #1

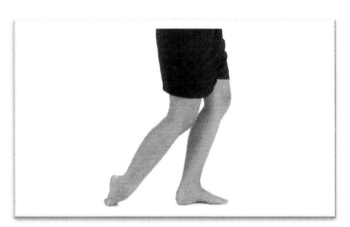

Stretch 1 – Foot-behind Shin Stretch:
Stand upright and place the top of your toes on the ground behind you. Push your ankle to the ground.

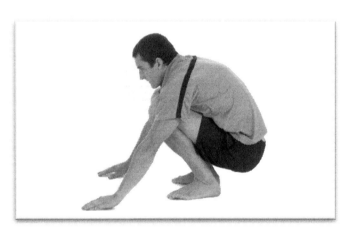

Stretch 2 – Squatting Achilles Stretch:
Stand with your feet shoulder width apart. Then bend your legs and lower your body into a sitting position. Place your hands out in front for balance.

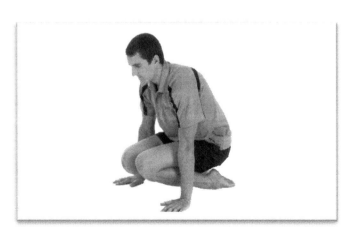

Stretch 3 – Double Kneeling Shin Stretch: Sit with your knees and feet flat on the ground. Sit back on your ankles and keep your knees together. Place your hands next to your knees and slowly lean backwards while raising your knees off the ground.

Stretching Routine for
Anterior Compartment Syndrome #2

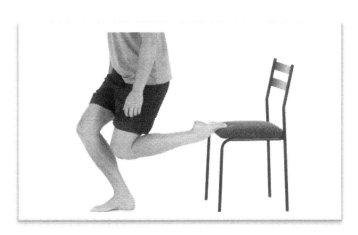

Stretch 1 – Raised Foot Shin Stretch:
Stand with your back to a chair. Place the top of your toes onto the chair and then push your ankle downwards.

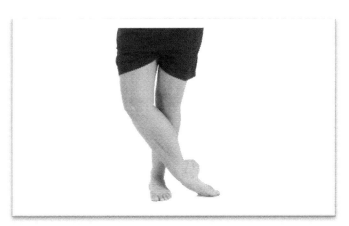

Stretch 2 – Front Cross-over Shin Stretch: Stand upright and place the top of your toes on the ground in front of your other foot. Slowly bend your other knee to force your ankle to the ground.

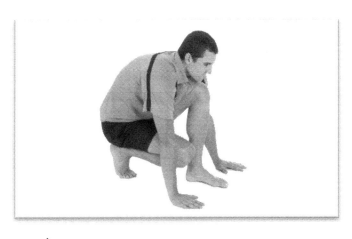

Stretch 3 – Squatting Toe Stretch: Kneel on one foot with your hands on the ground. Keep the toes of your rear foot on the ground, slowly lean forward and arch your foot.

Stretching Routine for Ankle Sprain #1

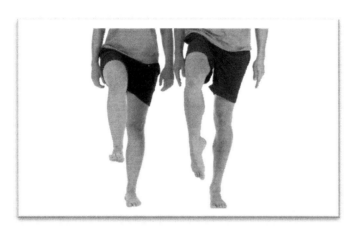

Stretch 1 – Ankle Rotation Stretch: Raise one foot off the ground and slowly rotate your foot and ankle in all directions.

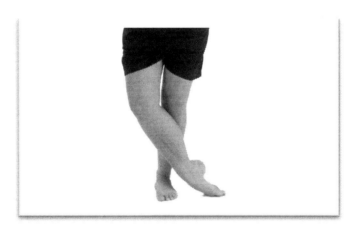

Stretch 2 – Front Cross-over Shin Stretch: Stand upright and place the top of your toes on the ground in front of your other foot. Slowly bend your other knee to force your ankle to the ground.

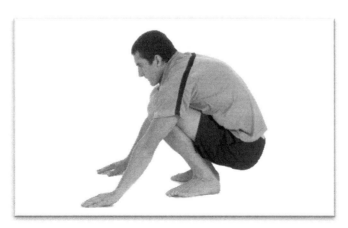

Stretch 3 – Squatting Achilles Stretch: Stand with your feet shoulder width apart. Then bend your legs and lower your body into a sitting position. Place your hands out in front for balance.

Stretching Routine for
Ankle Sprain #2

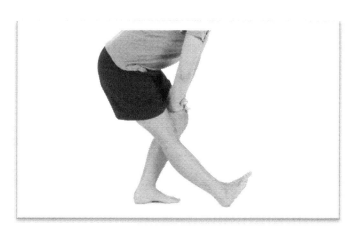

Stretch 1 – Standing Toe Raised Calf Stretch: Stand with one knee bent and the other leg straight out in front. Point your toes upwards and lean forward. Keep your back straight and rest your hands on your bent knee.

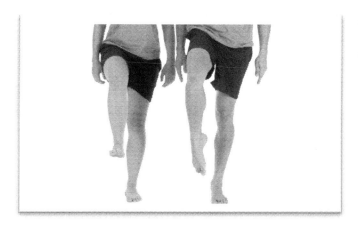

Stretch 2 – Ankle Rotation Stretch: Raise one foot off the ground and slowly rotate your foot and ankle in all directions.

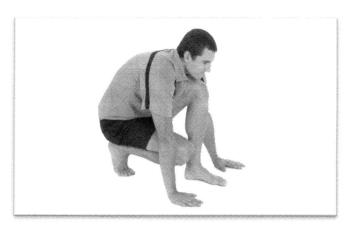

Stretch 3 – Squatting Toe Stretch: Kneel on one foot with your hands on the ground. Keep the toes of your rear foot on the ground, slowly lean forward and arch your foot.

Stretching Routine for
Posterior Tibial Tendinitis #1

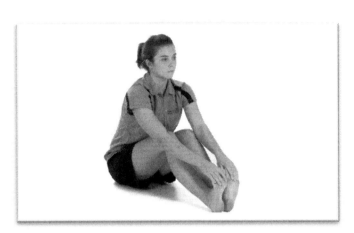

Stretch 1 – Sitting Toe-pull Achilles Stretch: Sit on the ground with your knees slightly bent. Hold onto your toes with your hands and pull your toes towards your body.

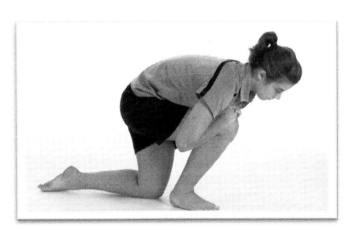

Stretch 2 – Kneeling Heel-down Achilles Stretch: Kneel on one foot and place your body weight over your knee. Keep your heel on the ground and lean forward.

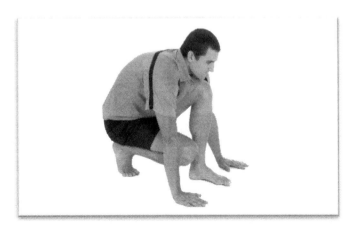

Stretch 3 – Squatting Toe Stretch: Kneel on one foot with your hands on the ground. Keep the toes of your rear foot on the ground, slowly lean forward and arch your foot.

Stretching Routine for Posterior Tibial Tendinitis #2

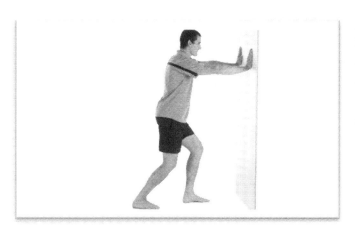

Stretch 1 – Leaning Heel-back Achilles Stretch: Reach towards a wall and place one foot as far from the wall as is comfortable. Make sure that both toes are pointing forward and your heels are on the ground. Bend your back knee and lean towards the wall.

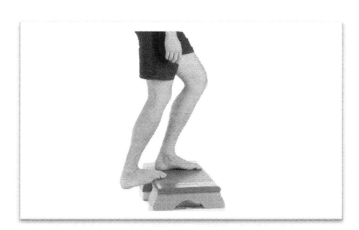

Stretch 2 – Single Heel-drop Achilles Stretch: Stand on a raised object or step and place the ball of one of your feet on the edge of the step. Bend your knee slightly and let your heel drop towards the ground.

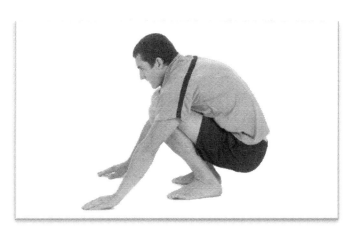

Stretch 3 – Squatting Achilles Stretch: Stand with your feet shoulder width apart. Then bend your legs and lower your body into a sitting position. Place your hands out in front for balance.

Stretching Routine for Peroneal Tendinitis #1

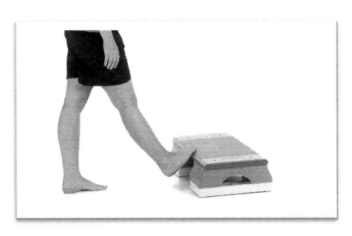

Stretch 1 – Standing Toe-up Calf Stretch: Stand upright and place the ball of your foot on a step or raised object. Turn your foot inward, keep your leg straight and lean towards your toes.

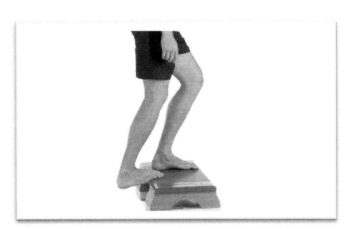

Stretch 2 – Single Heel-drop Achilles Stretch: Stand on a raised object or step and place the ball of one of your feet on the edge of the step. Turn your foot inward, bend your knee slightly and let your heel drop towards the ground.

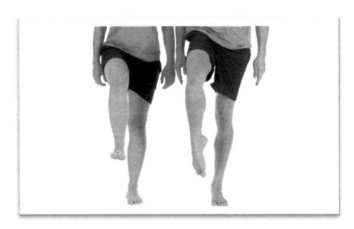

Stretch 3 – Ankle Rotation Stretch: Raise one foot off the ground and slowly rotate your foot and ankle in all directions.

Stretching Routine for Peroneal Tendinitis #2

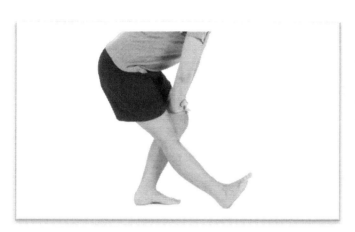

Stretch 1 – Standing Toe Raised Calf Stretch: Stand with one knee bent and the other leg straight out in front. Point your toes upwards and inward, and lean forward. Keep your back straight and rest your hands on your bent knee.

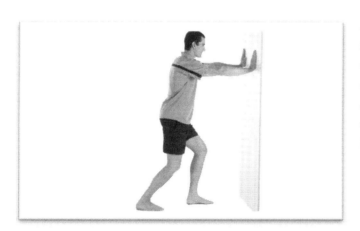

Stretch 2 – Leaning Heel-back Achilles Stretch: Reach towards a wall and place one foot as far from the wall as is comfortable. Make sure that both toes are pointing forward and your heels are on the ground. Bend your back knee and lean towards the wall.

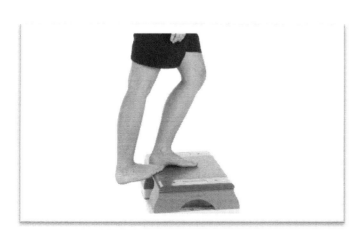

Stretch 3 – Single Heel-drop Calf Stretch: Stand on a raised object or step. Put the ball of one foot on the edge of the step, turn your foot inward and keep your leg straight. Let your heel drop towards the ground.

Stretching Routine for
Plantar Fasciitis #1

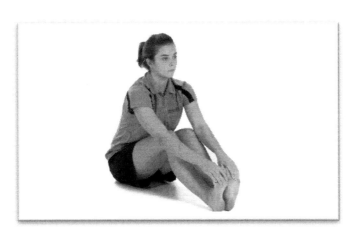

Stretch 1 –Sitting Toe-pull Achilles
Stretch: Sit on the ground with your knees slightly bent. Hold onto your toes with your hands and pull your toes towards your body.

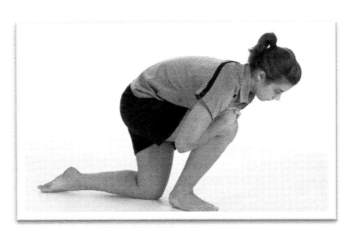

Stretch 2 – Kneeling Heel-down Achilles
Stretch: Kneel on one foot and place your body weight over your knee. Keep your heel on the ground and lean forward.

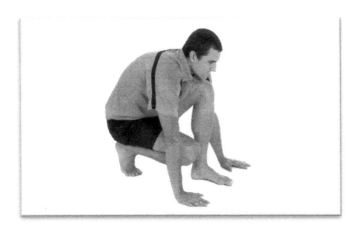

Stretch 3 – Squatting Toe Stretch: Kneel
on one foot with your hands on the ground. Keep the toes of your rear foot on the ground, slowly lean forward and arch your foot.

Stretching Routine for
Plantar Fasciitis #2

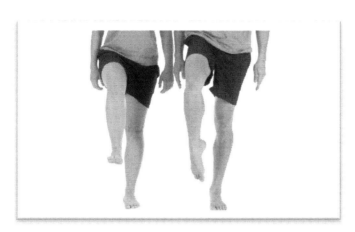

Stretch 1 – Ankle Rotation Stretch: Raise one foot off the ground and slowly rotate your foot and ankle in all directions.

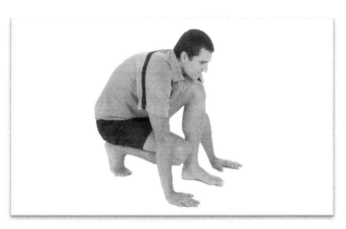

Stretch 2 – Squatting Toe Stretch: Kneel on one foot with your hands on the ground. Keep the toes of your rear foot on the ground, slowly lean forward and arch your foot.

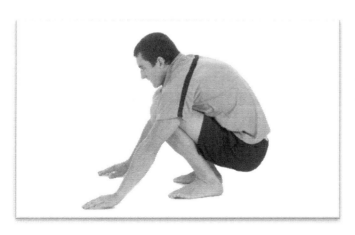

Stretch 3 – Squatting Achilles Stretch: Stand with your feet shoulder width apart. Then bend your legs and lower your body into a sitting position. Place your hands out in front for balance.